T0148376

Healthcare Solutions with Acupuncture

Gary F. Fleischman, OMD

Edited by
M. Carol Mihalik, MS

iUniverse, Inc.
New York   Bloomington

iUniverse books may be ordered through booksellers or by contacting:

iUniverse
1663 Liberty Drive
Bloomington, IN 47403
www.iuniverse.com
1-800-Authors (1-800-288-4677)

ISBN: 978-1-4401-3641-2 (sc)
ISBN: 978-1-4401-3642-9 (ebook)
ISBN: 978-1-4401-3643-6 (dj)

Printed in the United States of America

iUniverse rev. date: 6/4/2009

Dedicated to my sister Harlene Kravet whose continued encouragement has helped me to achieve my goals in life.

Foreword

The many health problems and health care costs facing our nation can be addressed by using methods suggested by Dr. Gary F. Fleischman in his book *Healthcare Solutions with Acupuncture*. He reviews many conditions that can be successfully treated and healed by acupuncture. Before he discusses various illnesses from A to W he explains the difference in Chinese medicine and compares it to the West. He was trained in a Chinese hospital. The practical and theoretical experiences in his training offer him an ability to evaluate the differences between Western and Eastern medicine.

He offers an explanation of the different medical sciences in acupuncture procedures and the comparison to surgery and use of drugs. The minimally invasive use of needles to treat minor and major illness could result in a tremendous reduction in health care costs for our nation. As we move towards more preventive medicine, acupuncture could be a solution to reduce costs spent on diagnostic procedures, drugs to treat illness and even surgery. Although acupuncture is not clearly understood by the general population of the United States, more people would be open to it after reading a good book on healthcare solutions using acupuncture. Many individuals may be happy to have a better understanding of how needles are used to achieve balance in the energy within the body.

Dr. Fleischman can help many individuals understand acupuncture through his explanation of the four medical subjects, which include anatomy, chemistry, microbiology, and psychology/psychiatry. This holistic explanation encourages many people to want to achieve a balance of body energy to resolve acute and chronic medical conditions. His solutions of a better way to address cause of disease, process of disease, Qi energy, diagnosis of disease, and treatment of disease, provide an understanding of how Eastern and Western Medicine differ. The holistic approach, including the emotional effects of illnesses, would lend itself to more acceptance by individuals.

The flow of energy, as he explains it, creates a way to follow the Yin-Yang principles of health. The wholesome longevity, of Chinese and Japanese medical care, which is related to diet and nutrition, would bring health to most Americans. Americans could learn from Dr. Fleischman's emphasis on Chinese and Japanese medicine.

Throughout the remaining chapters of his book, he selects various diseases and conditions and compares the approaches of the Western versus the Chinese medicine. His comparison to Western medicine clearly leaves one feeling that we in America must learn to apply the Eastern medical approach to medicine to reduce health care costs by using acupuncture.

It is great honor to write a foreword to a book that will become a required text in the Holistic Health Class taught at Southern Connecticut State University.

Doris M. Marino, PhD, MPH
Associate Professor and Coordinator of School Health Education
Southern Connecticut State University

Caveat

If you choose to use any health exercise or procedure described in this book, you should seek direction from a practitioner authoritative in the particular field.

Contents

Acknowledgments

Many have guided me in the teachings of Chinese medicine. Special appreciation of the knowledge I apply on paper goes to Dr. Ki-Kun Wan, my mentor and associate, who shared with me his Chinese medical and cultural wisdom. To Dr. Ralph Alan Dale, an outstanding instructor in acupuncture, and dear friend, to whom I'm grateful. At the China Institute of Acupuncture, many thanks to both Dr. James Gotcher and Dr. Hadi Kareem for their in-depth studies on Oriental medicine. To the staff of physicians at the Guangdong Provincial Hospital of Traditional Chinese Medicine, for providing me with invaluable clinical training in a hospital setting, xiexie.

In writing this book, much appreciation goes to my loyal friend G.F. for her computer expertise and to my nephew Scott Kravet for his very useful suggestions. I thank my patient and friend M. Carol Mihalik for her wonderful editorial abilities.

Introduction

Healthcare issues today encompass a wide range of increasing concerns such as availability, affordable cost, effective and safe procedures, the needs of children, and quality of life. Ways of improvement often appear outside modern mainstream medicine. Established inexpensive routines with proven results actually arise from ancient medical wisdom. Many can be found within the scope of Chinese medicine, and specifically acupuncture.

To serve the public competently, it's beneficial to focus on coexistence—even in proposed universal healthcare systems. Rather than merging and mixing medical principles where accurate diagnosis and treatment goals lose themselves, the old and the new require their separate standards of care with joint cooperation. *Healthcare Solutions with Acupuncture* holds the answers for the best we can offer our patients. This remains the book's purpose.

As a full practice of medicine that evaluates disease and treats the sick based on thousands of years of advancements, acupuncture methods are there for the taking. To gain an overall perception of its concepts, each part of the book provides easy to understand classifications of sickness, techniques of needling, and the healing process.

Throughout the chapters, you will see continual comparisons between Western and Chinese medicine. This format allows greater analysis of the unfamiliar by way of the familiar. Just from your personal experience in healthcare, you will achieve new depths of knowledge. Of course both types of science have much proven merit. But together, with respect for differences, better medical care will emerge. Better signifies more effective and less risky, and certainly less costly.

During my early years in a surgical specialty, I put time aside to study unconventional medical alternatives. Results seen from acupuncture greatly impressed me. I decided to pursue a goal of developing expertise in this field, with the realization that like surgery, learning diagnostic and dexterous skills was mandatory. A fifteen-year teacher-student association with a physician from Beijing was followed by the completion of Chinese medical courses and hospital training in China. This allowed me to earn a Doctorate in Oriental Medicine. I have applied and taught Traditional Chinese Medicine ever since.

Improved medicine will evolve when you understand what every healthcare professional has to offer. If drugs, surgery and your doctor's advice keep you healthy, stay with it. But if your choices do not prevent or heal disease, or maintain quality of life, look elsewhere.

My growing awareness and self-application of Chinese medicine truly has led me to attain a greater soundness of body and mind. Personally, my medical needs are fulfilled with Chinese herbal remedies, massage therapy, acupuncture and little else. I have combined lifestyle habits from Traditional Chinese Medicine together with Western natural medicine. Presently as a senior-citizen grandfather, I have never experienced a severe type of illness. Moreover, I have never been a patient in a hospital and I have never had flu shots or the flu. Throughout my adult life, I have never bought health insurance other than what's required of me for auto insurance.

Many of us hold loyalties to conventional medicine. Even if we read about a proven alternative method, we might disregard it in favor of the established drug prescription or surgery. We have confidence in our physician authority figure from childhood conditioning. Their recommendations to improve a condition, however, may just bring us to alternatives.

Yet numbers of citizens initially choose the more natural forms of care and prefer not to carry a lot of insurance. Unfortunately, as we well know, masses of people cannot afford any coverage at all, but they may be able to manage an acupuncture treatment.

Then there are groups who select from both, perhaps mainstream diagnostic procedures on one hand, and natural childbirth by a midwife on the other. Of course, emergency rooms can prevent fatalities. Though even here acupuncture procedures can make recoveries easier.

I discovered health secrets mainly through acupuncture's use of energy. My vocation in acupuncture helped me to develop this insight. Areas of health and disease can be understood in terms of Western Medicine's studies of structure (anatomy), chemistry, physiology, bacteria, viruses, and psychology as well as in terms of Oriental Medicine's concepts of invisible forces. Our responsibility to ourselves demands comprehensive knowledge, and the more initiative we take to help ourselves inexpensively, the less our need for extensive coverage from insurance companies. Of course, there is much controversy today over the profitable insurance industry's refusal to pay for all patient claims.

You will notice that several words begin with a capital letter. Ordinarily, Heat, Blood and Liver, for example, are written with small letters. Energy associations to the terms quite often take the designation by a capital. Whether in health or disease, the energy involvement is expressed in this way.

Chapter 1
Acupuncture Procedure

With needles in hand, each made of a solid pointed filament attached to a tiny oblong handle, acupuncturists attempt to correct health problems. Exact insertions are based on age-old medical principles. Needled patients enter a healing process; pleasant sensations of comfort and relaxation frequently arise. The body heals itself and alleviates the ailment. Routines of penetration, judgment of depth, and angling, adhere to procedures performed worldwide.

For thousands of years, the above application to pierce the skin and cure a disease has taken place in China. As the most populous country on the planet, filled with extremely active and hardy elderly, there must be connections between their wholesomeness and their way of healthcare. Traditional methods incorporate energy exercises, herbal medication, food therapy, massage therapy and acupuncture. Western countries continue to adopt these practices as we search for a healthier lifestyle. More and more practitioners from America and Europe take courses to develop skills needed to apply Chinese medicine.

From a conventional surgical-specialty background, I made a career change to Chinese medicine. Limitations on curing disease by surgery and drugs motivated me to explore other methods. When diplomatic relations were established in the early 1970s between the United States and China, media coverage revealed the Chinese way of life. Much attention focused on their medical establishments. It showed how huge numbers of the sick received means of help that differed from surgery and synthetic drugs. I thought that perhaps it had the answers I was looking for. I'm happy to say it did. Frequent news items at that time featured herbal remedies, traditional Chinese massage, and acupuncture, which became my special interest.

I read all I could on the subject and attended hard-to-find courses. In 1980, I invited a Chinese doctor from Beijing to join me in my practice as my acupuncture mentor. We agreed that I would provide him access to patients and he in turn would try to teach me everything he knew. It was a wonderful learning experience that lasted until 1995, when he retired. In addition to Chinese medicine, I gained a deeper appreciation of Chinese culture and language.

Acupuncture became very helpful in my practice, especially for the treatment of disabilities and vascular disorders. I became aware of Chinese medicine's understanding of disease and the effectiveness of acupuncture needling. This influenced me—even at an older age—to devote four years of my life pursuing a doctorate in Oriental Medicine. Hospital training was required in China. With a renewed dedication, I made a complete career change.

Compared To Surgery

Means by which surgery and acupuncture try to achieve desired results are comparable. Both use invasive techniques and both operate with sterile instruments. A scalpel blade secured to a usually flat handle grasped by the surgeon's fingers incises the skin. Other instruments may retract the opening to identify and reconstruct or maybe remove unwanted body parts.

In contrast, acupuncture goes through the skin with fingertips guiding thin needles to affect a therapeutic outcome. Surgery repairs structure in hopes of a better function. Acupuncture at first corrects function, and then afterwards a structural change may result. The scope of healing follows improvement in circulation, achieved by draining blockages and toxins and restoring nutrients to damaged tissue.

Surgeons have normal and abnormal anatomy in mind. A common operation for appendicitis consists of its immediate removal (appendectomy). Painful inflammation of the appendix (appendicitis) is a diseased structure that does not belong in a healthy body. Acupuncturists hold a mindset of healthy or dysfunctional body energy. Acupuncture regards appendicitis as a diseased condition, harmful to normal working energy. Called intestinal abscess, its cause comes from excess Heat and circulatory Stagnation. Treatment by needle insertions will clear the Heat and disperse the Stagnation.

The difference not only lies in treatment, but also in evaluation. In this case, Western medicine would diagnose inflammation in a certain body part. Chinese medicine would assess abnormal conditions in circulation and the internal environment as too much Stagnation and Heat.

Compared To Drugs

The pharmaceutical industry provides pills and tablets in various shapes and colors. From years of research, the chemical make-up of the drug and biochemical actions in the body become known. A person swallows a pill and the body responds—explainable by biochemistry.

Likewise, the insertion of an acupuncture needle also influences the body to react in a particular way. This response embodies invisible forces, polarities, energy and matter; in part the science of physics. But it also involves all invisible forces encountered by human beings to include circulatory functions, emotions and spiritual dimensions.

The word energy commonly describes this invisible power as well as the Chinese term Qi, pronounced chi or chee. It integrates with bodily structure and chemistry (anatomy and biochemistry). Physiology in Western medicine builds on chemistry; in Chinese medicine we have an energy physiology.

Say you walk down the street one bright and crisp day and notice a tree before you, branches waving with leaves fluttering. No human or any type of animal seems to be there to shake the tree. Suddenly you feel a cold sensation against your skin. What causes those branches to wave and those leaves to flutter? Obviously, it's the wind. Can you see the wind? Not at all, but you can feel the wind and see its actions on a very visible tree. This serves as an example of energy with three qualities: (1) it remains invisible, (2) it is perceived by touch and, (3) it acts on material objects. Chinese theory says energy can transform to matter, and matter to energy. To illustrate, picture a chunk of ice being heated in a pot on a stove. Soon the ice melts to water, and then rises as steam to become unseen vapors. Another example in Chinese medicine explains the body's extraction of energy from digested food and drink.

Diagnostic Procedure

A surgeon evaluates abnormal structures as seen by the naked eye and on X-rays, or from bits of tissue (biopsy) under a microscope; acupuncture evaluates energy from symptoms felt by patients. They sense abnormal energy. In addition to subjective descriptions of discomfort, examinations of the tongue, pulse, facial complexion, and behavior play a major role in acupuncture methods of disease interpretation. However, in treatment, both surgery and acupuncture use invasive techniques.

Diagnoses for drug prescriptions may entail laboratory tests such as blood chemistry and blood cell counts. Pharmaceuticals then treat the disorder by chemical means. Chinese medicine makes use of herbal medication, administered on principles of normal, abnormal, and blocked energy.

When someone comes to my office, I must evaluate accurately by consultation and physical examination to treat effectively. In general, a Western medical diagnosis from an initial exam also determines therapy, and added laboratory and X-ray information can prove helpful. The interpretation of symptoms by acupuncture calls for an energy diagnosis. For example, hypertension (high blood pressure) and migraine headaches are symptoms of Organ energy imbalances.

The majority of time during the initial visit is spent on the consultation, to assemble all the related facts. Abnormal energy is felt, so sensations described by the patient will give me valuable data. The more I understand the ailing experience, the better the care. I may need to know the effects of weather conditions, diet, food cravings, and stressful situations. If present, the type of pain, is it sharp, achy or burning?

Physical signs, seen or palpated, are often typified by inflammation and swelling. These confirm the symptoms with deeper recognition of the condition. The pulses—six on each wrist—and shape and color of the tongue reflect internal happenings. Facial complexion and personality also provide diagnostic information.

Often I am told that the source of a person's suffering cannot be found on MRI, by X-ray or laboratory tests. Western medicine will then conclude it's all in the mind. Actually, it may very well be in the energy systems, not seen by traditional diagnostic avenues.

Needle Procedure

Once I conclude the initial examination and evaluation, I decide on the best application for accurate needling. With a comprehensive understanding of energy movement that propels Blood circulation, added to the heart's pumping action that we know so well, I go to work. Acupuncturists think in terms of blocked energy and Stagnant Blood circulation, possibly with deficiencies or excesses and causes from negative emotions, all of which bring about disease. This may also be expressed in the body's anatomy, chemistry, and physiology.

While there may be a physiological response to single-needle stimulation, successful results occur with combinations of needles. One set of points corrects an illness that requires elimination of toxic Heat; another set restores normal circulation away from Stagnation and another taps into energy reserves.

My main concern centers on the best possible cure, while allowing a pleasant healing process. Proper manipulation of energy with proper instruments regenerates health. I gently insert the thin needles. So gently that many do not realize treatment has taken place. Some disorders though call for heavier stimulation, still

6

not painful. Automatically, the individual enters an altered state of relaxation, because the body cannot heal itself under stress. The body craves this healing and I am helping it do just that. Subtle music in the background offers additional means to relax the patient.

Each needle penetration consists of an operation unto itself to restore normalcy. Several approaches make themselves available such as the choice for a deep or superficial thrust, a light or heavy stimulation, or a perpendicular or angled direction. The method depends on the diagnosis. I hold the needle, fully aware that I will contact energy. Through this solid filament, I attempt to heal the ailment and choose the most beneficial operative technique.

My responsibility is to care for the sick and the affliction that disturbs the body's energy. We are dealing with complexities of life-sustaining vital forces. Illness stems from malfunction of these forces. Healing the energy brings recuperation. Methods with the needle provide the answer for a correction.

Though some fail to respond, about 90% of my treatments result in relief, after the first visit. Nevertheless, reinforcements are frequently necessary to thoroughly correct the ailment. While the initial evaluation is established by how the patient feels, follow-up progress is also based on subjective experience. Symptoms may recur in weeks, months or years later. Then the body will know how much acupuncture is needed. It responds to the effects of treatment.

Follow-up visits help attain greater levels of recovery in order to regain health. However, each session must have a reevaluation through interpretation of changes from discomfort to relief. Acupuncture is wonderfully flexible. Needle stimulation can be added or lessened depending on the patient's needs at the time. Some chronic conditions require maintenance care over a long period. But as a rule, pain decreases and strength increases as energy function improves.

Additional Help

Various modalities supplement needling. A number of decisions are kept in mind regarding the selection of acupuncture points and methods of insertion. Supplements heed further consideration. They must also meet the needs to heal the ailment.

Herbal heat, like needle instruments, dates back to China's antiquity. In fact, the Chinese term for acupuncture consists of two words, needle-heat. The main herbal substance is mugwort. It is usually called by its Japanese name, moxa. In countries outside of Eastern Asia, mugwort becomes a vegetative nuisance to be weeded out of the garden. China, on the other hand, cultivates, harvests, processes, packages and uses it for therapeutic heat. Intense heat with pleasant sensations penetrates through the skin for healing benefits. It treats as well as prevents disease.

I apply the medicinal warmth over certain points on myself almost everyday. My strong immunity, I believe, is attributed to this self-treatment and other practices. For example, I frequently give myself acupuncture needling, consume herbal medications and receive massage. However, no one should administer moxa without adequate training; it can cause bodily harm. The same caveat applies to all professionally established forms of Chinese medicine.

Another modality consists of suction cups. Based on an ancient procedure, a number of ethnic groups residing in Europe, Africa and America adopted and improved upon it. Originally a flame of fire heated the inside of an animal's horn to create a vacuum. In its primitive form, suction by mouth was used at the pointed tip opening.

While Western countries gradually stopped using suction types of therapy, Asia has perfected and expanded the method. Materials of bamboo, glass and plastic, today comprise the material for the cups. A Japanese innovation incorporates a suction pump, which offers a degree of control. Acupuncture clinics in Chinese hospitals routinely employ these vacuum methods.

Frequently seen in acupuncture offices are electrical machines with protected wires that clamp onto needles. The stimulation enhances the acupuncture effect. After an extended period there is desensitization. Acupuncture anesthesia works in this way. However, a shorter span of time regulates circulation, decreases pain and results in normal sensations.

As a student of Traditional Chinese Medicine, I lived in a Chinese hospital and trained intensely in the clinics. Writing extensive details of cases satisfied part of the doctorate requirements. I learned how routines of acupuncture needling commonly included suction cupping, electrical needle stimulation and heat. Most of the heat was provided by an infrared heat lamp, and less moxa. Actually, Japan treats more with moxa. Called moxibustion, in Japan two separate certifications exist, one for acupuncture and one for moxa. Acupuncturists, however, usually have both.

Chinese clinics prefer the bamboo cup, with heat procedure from a burning cotton ball soaked in alcohol. Due to breakage on hard floors, glass is generally not used. These clinics offer both inpatient and outpatient services. Many come for appointments from their homes. Large numbers are transported from their hospital beds. Furthermore, bedridden patients can receive treatment right in the wards or private rooms. A doctor goes from patient to patient with a wheeled cart carrying sterile needles, bamboo cups and all other necessary instruments and materials. Even in the most modern hospital setting, the effectiveness of centuries-old acupuncture techniques continues to be recognized.

Care of Patients' Energy

In my office, I use so much of what I learned from my Chinese hospital experience where patients accept and appreciate all therapies provided, and where nobody complains. Since routines have been proven, founded on thousands of years of progress, there are satisfying results and few complications. Of course, desired cure of disease does not always take place, but the rate of success stays high.

These medical achievements originate from a deep understanding of life-sustaining forces. Care for physical and emotional problems starts with energy networks. A complex dimension of the body serves as a basis of existence. It embraces inherited sources, the anatomy and the physiology, the mind and the spirit, which Chinese medical science holistically incorporates.

On my first day in the acupuncture clinics, I noticed a very young boy with a mental deficiency. I asked my supervising physician about the cause and treatment of the child's condition. In her scientific terms, she explained that the boy failed to completely inherit the spiritual energy (the souls) from the parents. Treatment consisted of special acupuncture needling in the head, palms and soles. I then observed an older doctor who specialized in this procedure; he did the acupuncture while mothers held their little ones in their laps. Following the insertions the children went to sleep and in time, additional treatments brought forth mental strengthening.

Another case involved a woman in her twenties who sustained injuries after being hit by a bus. As she reclined on a table face-up to receive acupuncture, her younger sister rested her head on the patient's abdomen. At a subsequent visit with improvement, I told the patient in Chinese that her sister loves her. She smiled to me knowing how this contact helps.

A man was washing his wife's laundry in a sink in a hospital ward. From her bed, she felt comfort and security as seen in her facial expression. He left the room for awhile to hang the clothes. Upon his return you could see the happiness of caring. I also saw family devotion as a daughter helped a nurse bathe her mother. In China, hospitals are receptive to family affection and participation in patient care.

Energy comes in different types. There's inherited energy that must last a lifetime. It cannot be replaced but it can be nourished and strengthened to aid problems, like the little boy born with inadequate intelligence. Another type, called acquired energy, needs replacement every day. This we get from what we eat, drink and breathe.

Energy enhancement in times of sickness becomes available from therapies such as acupuncture, herbal medication, diet and massage—further supplemented by the care and love we give to one another, like I saw in the Chinese hospital. Again and again I observe the value of family involvement that helps correct disorders.

An additional area of care for patients' energy directly centers on the doctor-patient relationship. Chinese medicine emphasizes the feelings of a person, followed by some physical examinations. In contrast, Western medicine's main goal is to determine the presence or absence of abnormal structures or function via X-ray pictures, scans, biopsies and many kinds of invasive scopes, plus laboratory tests of blood, blood cells and various body fluids.

Professional care of someone's energy, however, requires sensitivity to that person's self-description of symptoms. Because

11

energy is felt, not seen, and yet integrates into anatomy and body chemistry, a practitioner of Chinese medicine concentrates on and then evaluates the disturbances of vital forces. Nevertheless, a series of clinical treatments could become a matter-of-fact routine. Taught from my medical background, I used a bedside manner to assure comfort during therapy. To my surprise, the Chinese patients often requested the "American" doctor.

The hospital clinics consisted of large rooms with men and women of all ages lying flat on tables, reclining or seated. Privacy was not an issue. Overall, I have found that in China and back home in the States, relaxed comfort during treatment in any setting, works well.

Supervising physicians instructed me in terms of energy. An angled needle insertion toward a leg disability meant Qi transference would strengthen and rehabilitate the leg problem. Diagnosis reflected a number of different disorders in circulation of Qi such as Stagnation, Blockages, Cold or Heat, Deficiencies and Excesses. Organs come into play for assessment with knowledge of Organ forces. Diabetes, for example, previously was called "wasting thirsting disease". Then the name changed to "sweet urine disease". The terms designate signs and symptoms, but it truly fits into a disease syndrome of too much internal Heat. This relates to the energy aspect of Kidney that affects urination, Stomach that affects metabolism or Lung that affects thirst. In other words, what someone experiences follows a disease pattern with Organ connections. Trouble in energy, whether of the Organ or of far-reaching Channels, remains the source of the problem.

Patients' Choice

America and other Western democracies allow citizens to elect candidates for public office. In contrast, China provides government-appointed national and regional leaders. Medicine is an entirely different story. Whereas we have primary care physicians to coordinate healthcare according to needs and insurance plans, in China, patients make their own choices. A national health plan requires a co-payment for each visit in a selected clinic and the government pays the balance.

Every available heath service from acupuncture and herbal medicine to Western surgery can be had. Likewise, there are many Americans who prefer a personal option for their healthcare, thus the popularity of holistic medical choices.

My feelings predict more democracy in Chinese politics and more democracy in American medicine. This will result in the ability to vote for nominated candidates and to make healthcare decisions. In China, people are their own primary care physician, except in a crisis.

To understand how someone selects a field of medicine in China, we must understand the public's familiarity of accessible treatments and their indications. An ailing person enters a hospital and takes an elevator to a floor that would best care for his or her problem. Selections include herbs, acupuncture, massage, Western drugs and surgery. Upon leaving the elevator, one sees photos of doctors on the wall, with descriptions of their credentials placed under each picture. Now the sick individual picks a specific practitioner. At any time patients can change to, or add a different type of therapy. This is entirely their choice.

There are many hospitals that lean toward Western technique. Still, no matter how Western-oriented the hospital, by Chinese law it must have an acupuncture department. Patients can always fall back on the mother medicine when newer techniques prove ineffective or harmful. Repeatedly, I saw surgical complications treated by acupuncture.

The medical center, in which I trained, cared for about seven thousand patients a day. Well-equipped in surgery, obstetrics, diagnostic X-ray and an intensive care unit, thousands of patients received acupuncture daily, both inpatient and outpatient. The same large numbers were also given herbal drugs, orally and by injection, and massage therapy. From this multitude of patients, per day, only two or three had surgery. We can conclude that certain disorders operated upon with surgery in Western hospitals are treated through other methods in China. These would include acupuncture, herbal remedies taken by mouth, injected, or applied as therapeutic heat, and massage techniques.

Hospitals run herbal pharmacies with prescriptions from the internal medicine clinic. Every neighborhood also has a pharmacy. On the street, a person may visit and discuss symptoms with an herbal practitioner, followed by a medicinal recommendation for purchase. No middleman, it's between the patient and herbalist. On a personal note, part of my daily routine involves the intake of Chinese herbs. As soon as I became settled in my Chinese hospital guest-doctor room, I went to the corner herbal pharmacy and was able to buy the same herbal products I use back home.

An important medical specialty, with its own clinics and physicians, focuses on massage therapy. Performed by doctors who also interpret X-rays and lab tests when needed, it offers health services to masses of people in the hospital. Expertise has developed in subspecialties. I spent time with a doctor of massage who treated only infants and young children. Western skills concentrate mainly on anatomy and functions of nerves, muscles and joints. A major difference is that Chinese massage very much uses the same energy systems in practice as acupuncture. Today, many massage schools outside Asia do teach principles of energy and specific techniques known in Chinese as Tui Na or An Mo.

The Instrument

Instruments are an extension of the hands. Often the hand itself serves as an instrument, exemplified by massage and diagnostic palpitation. Trends in medicine always look for improved instrumentation. I remember when limited devices for examination consisted of the stethoscope, a scope to look into the ear or eye, percussion hammer, a basic X-ray machine, and laboratory tests performed by hand. Advancements brought us technology of MRI, scans, and body fluid analysis by automated instruments. Pharmaceutical research has refined medicinal substances and better ways to administer drugs. Organ transplants, laser and modified operations performed through small openings in the skin, illustrate surgical progress.

I often inspect my instruments, my acupuncture needles. Their invention and development impresses me as highly ingenious. Thousands of years ago someone realized that the stimulus from a pointed implement would result in a therapeutic reaction by the body. Primitive needles, carved from stone, progressed to bamboo shoots and sharpened pieces of bone, then molded from metal. Various designs and sizes meet the needs of application. For particular effects, needles absorb and direct moxa heat or electrical currents.

The true intellectual ability stems from energy principles of Chinese medical science. Surgeons operate through the knowledge of anatomy, sterile technique, and wound healing; internists prescribe drugs through their understanding of biochemistry; and acupuncturists insert disease-curing needles by their substantial comprehension of energy systems. It is the "science" of energy systems.

Chapter 2
A Different Medical Science

People often ask me whether or not I believe in various fields of medicine. Well, I believe in what works to correct an ailment and cause no harm. If a type of drug or procedure helps you to stay healthy and live a quality life, by all means stay with it. On the other hand, if your choice of therapy fails to provide you the wholesome life you so desire, look elsewhere.

When making comparisons between health services, it is best to seek information from practitioners who use the modality in question. Science is a system of knowledge. However, different systems embody different facts and principles. Confusion arises when one branch of established learning tries to interpret another. Indeed, acupuncture and Western medicine are worlds apart, emerging from dissimilar discoveries.

Consider a thoroughly experienced truck driver, whose only vehicle he has ever operated throughout his life, is his truck. His expertise to maneuver it as well or better than any other trucker comes from years on the job. He knows the workings of all the

17

intricate mechanical parts and has the ability to assess and repair any problem on the road. In spite of his comprehensive knowledge and trucking expertise, I do not think he is best suited to instruct a pilot on how to fly an airplane.

I also do not think a doctor without training or experience in acupuncture can explain acupuncture. Attempted rationale according to Western medical science, instead of Chinese medical science, falls into error. But what is the difference between the two sciences?

All fields of medicine have helped the sick, but all fields of medicine have had their setbacks. Some perform better in certain specialized areas. Plastic surgery does wonders in cosmetic repair. Acupuncture can, in many cases, reverse degenerative diseases. Outcome usually depends on what the doctor has to work with regarding the condition of the patient.

Both Western and Chinese methods do save lives. For awhile, a paramedic was my student, who had interest in using acupuncture lifesaving methods in the ambulance. His background training equipped him with the most updated technology of patient care in crisis medicine. Western understanding of human anatomy and physiology attends to urgent situations and often prevents fatality. However, when allowed, treatment on a patient's energy level with acupuncture has much to offer in life-and-death situations. This is only one example that shows improved health service when two types of medicine are performed together.

An available acupuncture guide for emergencies is published in Chinese and English. Titled *A Handbook for Treatment of Acute Syndromes by Using Acupuncture and Moxibustion,* the author, Prof. Mingqing Zhu has been invited as an honored lecturer to various countries. Saving of lives deserves every conceivable method. Both Western and Chinese medicine have much to offer.

Although they can be applied jointly, a big distinction between the two is understood by the words subjective and objective. The former relates to what patients feel, the latter to what doctors see. Acupuncture leans more toward the experience of the sick, frequently using tongue and pulse examinations to decide on treatment. Western medicine emphasizes the patient history, X-ray and laboratory reports, and physical findings to support a diagnosis. Thus, Chinese medicine is more subjective, Western medicine more objective.

Four Medical Subjects

Certain academic studies move in the same direction through the generations. We are therefore a reflection of our cultural and scientific heritage. Discoveries and new technology have advanced health routines, but the general ways of thinking remain unchanged. In Western medicine, I observe four basic divisions—four scientific subjects: anatomy, chemistry, microbiology, and psychology/psychiatry.

Anatomy

One deals with body structure, thoroughly dissected to know separate parts, inside and out. This is anatomy. Beyond normal anatomy, a field evolved to study abnormal anatomy, called pathology.

In three thousand years of Western civilization, superficial surgeries were performed to drain abscesses, repair military lacerations, and the like. Care was given for broken bones. However, the desired ability to do in-depth operations with in-depth knowledge of human anatomy, occupied historical medical minds. The Renaissance artist,

Leonardo Da Vinci, in the fifteenth century, completed hundreds of accurate drawings from his cadaver dissections. This served as a turning point. By the twentieth century, with pain and infection control, and anatomical insight, advanced surgical achievements appeared. Developments continue with innovative operations.

The invention of the microscope revealed observations of cellular anatomy. Centuries of labeling dissected material has given us a deep understanding of both normal and abnormal human tissue, seen by the naked eye and, with minute detail, through a microscopic lens. What the microscope disclosed, truly new-age knowledge, revolutionized medicine in Western countries. We continue to examine structure of cells and tissues in all dimensions, sizes, and conditions. We explore and hope to find answers to reverse degenerative disorders and cure tumors.

We apply our visual medicine for diagnosis and treatment with unlimited application. Professionals look into the body through X-ray and various scope instruments. The availability of these instruments led to less exploratory surgery. However, pathological studies of removed organs and biopsies do continue. Corrective surgery, chiropractic, and physical therapy fit this category of structure. It all relates to objective searching, examination, and correction directly on body parts that can be seen.

Chemistry

The science of physiology studies activities in cells and tissues. It attends to chemical and physical functions in living anatomy, mainly chemistry or the chemistry of life called biochemistry. Part of the science studies pressures of the heart and associated vessels plus nerve and brain energies and sound waves transmitted to the ear. But overall, the physiology is a physiology of body chemistry. There must be particles and matter as a rule. This concept will have more importance when compared to the physiology as understood in acupuncture.

So much of our medicine deals with the science of chemistry in two significant areas. One concerns medical laboratory testing of substances such as blood, urine, and spinal fluid. Done both for diagnosis and patient progress, doctors greatly depend on findings to determine treatments. The other serves as the basis for the pharmaceutical industry. Research leads to the formulation of drugs to be manufactured and packaged. A complete understanding of bodily chemical reactions and unwanted side effects produced by drugs, furnish the premise for the prescription.

Microbiology

Bacteria, viruses, and parasites have occupied much of Western medicine's investigations during the past two centuries. Studies conclude that these microorganisms hold the answers to causes and cures of many diseases. Thanks to the microscope, which also gave us the ability to closely examine cellular anatomy, we can now more fully comprehend the infectious process.

Antibiotics became a dominant class of drugs after World War II, dispensed by us ever since. As antibiotics lose their effectiveness over time, new generations of drugs are developed. Of course, viral conditions are another story. Viruses do not respond to antibiotics as do bacteria, but antiviral drugs have become available. Nevertheless, the attitude toward killing an "enemy" bug remains the same. Find and identify the pathogen, then find a means to destroy it, to cure the problem.

Through microscopic research, Western medical science advances. The search continues in pathologic structure, abnormal

21

physiology, and disease-producing microscopic life forms. This sets a significant direction on which future findings for better health will surface.

Psychology and Psychiatry

Behavioral sciences, in general, developed separately from other specialties. Psychology evaluates, and treats the mind and behavior, with consultation. As a medical specialty, psychiatry also employs drugs and surgery. Some chemistry overlap exists as specific psychiatric disorders show changes in the blood and metabolism. Ongoing findings demonstrate correlation between emotions and organ dysfunction, in other words, psychiatry can interact with internal medicine.

Western culture has its own general ideas about what's "all in the mind". This plays a part in diagnosis and therapy. Often when X-ray studies and laboratory test results reveal nothing wrong with a patient, who continues to experience discomfort, doctors conclude that it must be imagined—it must be psychological.

A seventeenth-century French philosopher, physicist, and mathematician by the name of René Descartes, strongly influenced Western science and attitudes. His famous quote states "I think, therefore I am". Accordingly, it must be all in the mind. In civilizations, East to West, history often reveals the source of massive influence, from which one person interprets existence.

Handling mental illnesses as separate entities led to the building of huge and numerous psychiatric institutions. Of course, patients require attention for physical problems, but therapy concentrates on mental and emotional disorders. Historic goals of psychiatry were to improve methods of care and move away from the harsh approaches meted out to those so afflicted.

Structure, Chemistry, Microbiology, Psychology/Psychiatry, and Acupuncture

Throughout the world, unique ways of looking at health, disease, and therapies evolve. Differences arise, even in bordering countries, even in bordering states in America. Practices of medicine pursue specific directions to reach various goals. The surgical direction progresses to perform procedures with less pain and decreased complications of infection. Pharmaceutical research invests millions of dollars to find and synthesize new and more effective drugs, to eliminate disease-producing bacteria or sedate anxiety. Diagnostic radiology invents equipment for more accurate visualization. And it all goes on endlessly.

Has acupuncture achieved its goals? It did, about two thousand years ago. The scientific principles were established to diagnose and understand the process of disease and a person's reactions to needle stimulation. This process of disease has much to do with circulatory disturbances, from prolonged negative emotions or harmful body invasions such as Damp Heat.

Written down in the world's oldest medical book, *The Yellow Emperor's Classic of Internal Medicine* continues as a major reference. Through the centuries no changes occurred in the basic teachings. Additional information through findings of prominent Asian physicians has broadened the application.

I group divisions of Western medicine into four general categories. This was done to understand connections with acupuncture and Chinese medicine. One word explains anatomy, biochemistry, microbiology and psychology/psychiatry in relationship to acupuncture: integration. What integrates everything in living human bodies is Qi energy. Energized force like blowing wind will be felt but not seen. It ties in with visible cell functions, actions of hormones, digestion, media to sustain bacteria, and behavior. We do not see energy, but we see and feel physical outcomes from the workings of energy. The Chinese concept of Qi energy, since antiquity, is defined as many universal forces encountered by humanity. In the Chinese vernacular, weather is heaven Qi, anger is Qi, a car is a Qi vehicle, since it runs by vapors.

Some years ago a breakthrough was made in the detection of Qi energy in a person. The discovery revealed that the lack of Qi permitted more electrical flow through a body part. Hence, increased Qi impeded the current. As a result, instruments were designed for measurement of energy and acupuncture point location.

As health professionals in Western Civilization pursued studies of visible body parts and their afflictions, Chinese doctors concentrated on the invisible power behind what was observed. They recognized functional energy patterns in health and disease. For instance, harmony in opposites (Yin and Yang) means well being. In contrast, imbalance produces illness.

All of existence divides into connected pairs of contrast—health and disease included. Cold and Hot serves as an example of a Yin-Yang partnership. Too much Cold Yin in the presence of inadequate Warm Yang will result in a Cold Sickness. Likewise, the opposite holds true when abundant Yang gives rise to a Hot Disease. Other Yin-Yang pairs include Damp-Dry, Stagnant-Rousing and Deficient-Excess. Unhealthy imbalances can happen in all four categories of Western Medicine.

Anatomy and Acupuncture

Structural studies of the human body play a dominant role in Western Medicine. For better understanding of anatomy, divisions of the subject were conceived to illustrate finer distinctions. Gross anatomy refers to that observed by the naked eye. Microscopic anatomy probes into two further divisions of (1) tissues and, (2) cells. We find specialized areas of embryo and fetal development. Bones, joints, and muscles are extensively labeled, as are nerves, sense organs, and the skin itself. These structures and organs take a place in related body systems such as nerves and the nervous system; the heart and the cardiovascular system; the lungs and the respiratory system; the stomach, intestine, liver, gallbladder and the digestive system; the kidneys, urinary bladder, reproductive organs and the urogenital system. There are also endocrine glands like the thyroid and adrenals.

A lot of terms identify body parts, large and small. The medical subject of anatomy was deemed so important in the past, students memorized passages from Gray's Anatomy. In some schools they still do. Orientation emphasizes that if you know your anatomy, you know your medicine. Compare that way of thinking with Chinese Medicine's premise to know your energy is to know your medicine.

Diseased anatomy brings us to the subject of pathology, with great interest in cellular pathology. By examining the abnormal side by side with the normal, illness in terms of human form becomes understood. During my residency, and when time permitted, I would follow surgical excisions to the pathology department. There to gain a deeper understanding of the patient's condition, I would examine the diseased tissue and the prepared slides under the microscope.

Acupuncture relates to anatomy and pathology in a different way. Within cells, tissues and other structures, vital forces dwell or circulate. If energy functions properly, anatomy stays healthy on gross and cellular levels. However, energy Stagnation, deficiency and afflictions with toxins or pathogenic elements, will result in pathology. Toxins occur with infection. Pathogenic elements include abnormal Heat, Cold, Dryness, and Dampness.

Procedures to harvest organs need maintenance energy from the donor and revitalizing energy from the recipient. It is an operation done in a limited time span. Once removed, the life-sustaining force gradually dwindles.

In general, integrated essential vital energy gives life to the physical human being. Disturbances to somebody's internal forces will produce unhealthy changes in structure. Impairment to one can disrupt the other at the same time. Life functions of Organs, tissues and Blood circulation depend on energy partnerships. As the body and its energy separate, life subsides. Life ceases when the partnerships break up.

Treatment of sick energy, with the associated sick-body area, uses acupuncture for both. At first, I reach an assessment by way of questions and examination. Laboratory and X-ray results are very informative. However, Chinese diagnostic methods—tongue, pulse, and palpitation—more closely direct an acupuncture treatment. Detection of Stagnation or Dampness for example, requires traditional Chinese insight. In turn, established principles of indicated needling frequently correct the problem.

Although my main mode of therapy centers on acupuncture, other practices of Oriental Medicine incorporate the same medical standards, based on workings of energy. These consist of herbal medicine and massage therapy (a medical specialty performed by physicians). We diagnose through energy dysfunction and treat by manipulating energy. Acupuncture needle stimulation elicits a physiological response, perhaps to activate Stagnant Blood and energy or resolve Dampness. Effective treatment concentrates on knowledge of expected reactions to specific needling.

In summary, energy integrates throughout all forms of anatomy. Disruption in the invisible Qi energy dimension will impair physical body parts. Affliction to one damages the other simultaneously. Vital activities of Organs as well as Blood circulation survive on energy relationships. When separated, degeneration sets in.

Biochemistry and Acupuncture

Western physiology, defined as the science of life in the body, explores and documents biochemical and physical functions. The basis of acupuncture, in comparison, follows energy physiology. And yet, Western medicine has acknowledged energy in areas such as metabolic production of calories, movement of fluids around cells, and of blood flow from the heart's pumping mechanism. Energy also contracts muscle fibers.

What is the difference between energies as understood by Western medicine and Chinese medicine? Well, the former must accurately measure substance and physical movements as part of the science. The pure energy studies of the latter interpret conditions with approximation, i.e., too much Cold, or deficient Blood.

I readily choose the words chemistry and biochemistry to explain physiology of Western medicine, since chemical actions deal with a large part of the subject. They even underlie several physical activities. Nerve-muscle stimulation for contraction, by a neurotransmitter, serves as an example.

For purposes of comparison, major chemical applications in Western medicine, evaluation and treatment, rely on diagnostic laboratory tests and pharmaceuticals. It must be understood that acupuncture looks at normal and abnormal body functions in terms of balanced or disrupted energy. In addition, diagnosis and therapy depend on conditions in these invisible forces.

Energy physiology, like conventional physiology, is the science of life. Instead of chemical and physical exploration and documentation, it studies energy. There are comparable observations, however, to clarify the scientific knowledge in each. Western science employs a distinct word to define internal-maintenance balance among glandular secretions and biochemical exchanges on the cellular level. The word is homeostasis. Chinese medicine has paired qualities with opposite features called the Yin and the Yang. This explains universal harmonies and disharmonies with much relevance to health and disease. All aspects of acupuncture are based on principles of connected contrasts as in dampness (Yin) to dryness (Yang) and deficiency (Yin) to excess (Yang).

Details of how the heart pumps blood and how the lungs oxygenate it, and the kidneys regulate it, comprise many physical and chemical processes in Western medical subjects. Components of blood, such as blood cells, have significance in diagnosis. The Chinese concept of circulation involves a Yin-Yang of Blood-energy relationship. Blood houses energy, which in turn propels Blood.

Whereas Western medicine takes into account hormonal production from organs, Chinese medicine concentrates on energy output in an integrating Organ sequence. Besides blood flow, Western physiology understands the flow or conduction of nerve impulses. The Chinese concept of energy flow embodies a complex of connecting Channels that penetrate the entire body. This encompassing network vitalizes Organs, tissues, Blood, nerves and all the physical and chemical actions.

Microbiology and Acupuncture

Tiny disease-producing organisms have attracted much attention in Western Civilization, ever since in-depth studies began in the eighteen hundreds. Many diseases are the result of bacteria, viruses, parasites, and fungi, whose presence has been explored and documented. These significant discoveries were made possible by microscopic research. Microbiology holds thorough explanations for infection based on these intricate observations. Medical practitioners at first identify the microorganism. Then the indicated medication, often an antibiotic, attempts to eradicate the culprit.

Chinese medicine operates with a different and much older approach. Since ancient times, doctors have recognized toxins as part of the infectious process. In addition, pathogenic elements in forms of Heat and Dampness contribute to the problem. A weak immune system does not help much either. These factors, of course, support sickness-related germs. The focus of treatment aims to restore a healthy internal environment, in which infectious organisms cannot survive. Acupuncture or herbal medication or both usually achieve results. Chinese medicine finds the problem within the surroundings of an unhealthy interior, which may harbor microbes; Western medicine focuses on the microbe itself.

Psychology/Psychiatry and Acupuncture

Unlike Western medicine, Chinese medicine never separated mental and emotional disorders from respiratory, digestive, urinary, and other physical problems. Emotions themselves act as invisible forces or types of energy. These feelings, when ailing, are subjective symptoms to be placed in a diagnostic evaluation.

Acupuncture treats psychological sickness in the same way it treats physical problems, by needle insertion. The stimulation causes a physiological response to heal the body and mind. It's amazing to our way of thinking that an identical needle application can take care of fatigue, loss of voice, and fever as well as insanity, depression, and hysteria. I use the same point for low back pain as I do, when needed, for anxiety.

Some people mistakenly regard acupuncture in terms of suggestion or on a "must believe in it for it to work" premise. Well, it's not a placebo. The needles do their job whether you believe in it or not. Many of my patients display both physical and mental ailments and several patients only have disturbances of just their body or just their psyche. Either way, I see effective results even among the strongest skeptics.

Disorders stem from various sources. A chief causative factor for a very large number of diseases has been known to arise from prolonged negative emotions. This phenomenon has remained rooted in the principles of Chinese medicine for so long that practitioners know with complete understanding what specific emotional problems relate to what specific physical problems.

Emotions one experiences become evident through a person's self-awareness. I often ask a patient what is felt under stress. A description of depression or worry will often match the physical complaint. Based on this information, effective acupuncture treats both.

Chapter 3
A Better Way

Health care concerns continue to escalate along a spectrum of issues. Affordable drugs for all ages and cures for degenerative diseases are but a few. When candidates run for political office, they advocate for reform in payment coverage or selected medical studies as in stem cell research. Medical bills are not a problem for the very wealthy nor sickness for the very healthy. There are those who never or rarely become patients in a hospital and, by choice, never buy health insurance. However, solutions are needed for people with budget difficulties who suffer from illness. Insurance premium expenses also burden employers responsible for their employees, as well as the employees themselves, with limitations in coverage, co-payments and deductibles.

We are repeatedly reminded that among the industrial nations, the United States incurs the highest health care costs, and yet, we are not the healthiest people. It does not make sense. We should be the healthiest. True, groups of elderly have attained older age,

31

methods have been found to reverse several fatal diseases, but many serious maladies have yet to receive corrective means.

Does effective treatment exist for all sicknesses? I sincerely think so. It's a matter of taking a different approach. The answer can be uncovered by your choices for health. When medical guidelines include every possible proven resource, without limitation, help is on the way.

While studying acupuncture in a Chinese hospital, I found many established clinics. Of course, Traditional Chinese Medicine was most in demand with its acupuncture, massage therapy, and herbal medication. Besides taken by mouth, herbs were also administered by injection directly into an acupuncture point. Processing the substance allowed this, also by intravenous (IV) intake. Imagine! They use herbal IV therapy. Other facilities included surgery, an intensive care unit (ICU), obstetrics and various other Western medical services. Healthcare becomes complete through the availability of every service possible. Thus modern facilities should still incorporate acupuncture. One can always turn to traditional medicine in case of poor results with other modalities.

Standards of living in all countries reflect original social developments. This applies to medicine as well. To provide the best care for our population, we borrow from each other as demonstrated by China's adoption of an intravenous drip to administer their herbal remedies.

The country with the oldest male and female residents in the world proves to be Japan. Writings on the subject emphasize a diet of fish, green tea, and miso soup. Overlooked are therapies such as an energy massage technique called shiatsu and a refined acupuncture routine with unique methods of insertion. Their profession of herbal medicine was modified from the Chinese. These changes offer remarkable benefit to many Japanese and to others.

More and more, America and Europe are looking into each Eastern culture and adopting the ways taught by ancient wisdom to maintain a wholesome life.

Fields other than acupuncture, herbs and massage do operate with Chinese medical principles, namely Qi exercises called Tai Chi Chuan and Qigong. Some Western professionals actually incorporate a few of the basics in bodywork and psychotherapy.

A concept to blend alternative practice into mainstream health care gave us the expression "Complementary and Alternative Medicine" (CAM). Complementary services enhance the basic treatment to make it more complete. The alternative will substitute a different form of therapy. Many regard these as simple modalities, when in fact they frequently consist of autonomous vocations to evaluate, treat and prevent illness. A plan where the professions work together is by coexistence. Each governs its own standards of care, without confusion or mishap in combined therapies. Harm does happen. Gentle acupuncture rehabilitation can be undone due to forceful therapies from a different kind of service.

A better way to health and longevity comes via information from the experiences of the very fit. What gives them soundness of body and mind? Their routines may show us how to be not only therapeutically effective, but less expensive too. I'm always on the lookout for time-tested means of personal well being. From extensive reading, courses and even from my patients, I learn a lot. Obviously, my main interest dwells in Oriental medicine, but with devoted attention to our natural medicine. As you make comparisons to our conventional medicine, you will understand all these holistic approaches.

Cause of Disease

A statement commonly found in Western medical textbooks reads "etiology unknown". This means the cause of the disease remains undiscovered. Known origins, however, fall into a list that includes categories of organ dysfunction, infection, chemical imbalance, ingested toxins, injuries, insect and animal bites, weak immunity, nutritional deficiencies, tissue degeneration, psychological sources, and inherited or congenital (present at birth) defects. One cause could complicate another. A laceration could become an infected wound, resulting from general weak immunity.

Areas of agreement exist between the two medical sciences. Acupuncture recognizes the above but with necessary additions for a thorough assessment of every etiology. The additions consist of disease-producing forces that disrupt normal body energy.

Behind the physical and biochemical disorders of organs, lies disturbed energy. The reverse also holds true. Tissue injury obstructs circulating energy and infection contaminates energy with toxins. In essence, pathogenic forces damage a human's vital powers, which could create extensive physical problems. Comprehending the nature of the disease-producing elements will explain the disease process.

Historically, China's insights into illness revealed causative factors that generated serious problems. Based in the detrimental effect of ongoing negative emotions, we can grasp the formation of problems. Stress for a day or so, easily put in the back of mind, poses no danger. Rather, it is the prolonged thought-provoking problems we dwell on week after week, month after month, keeping us awake at night. This can lead to threatening disorders.

Emotions develop within us, yet another etiology category

concerns elements that invade from outside of us. In destructive form, Wind, Heat, Cold, and Damp enter the body to produce illness. They may carry and provide a supportive media for bacteria and viruses, however, acupuncture focuses on the media.

When we become aware of the various sources of disease, ways of prevention come to light. Also, with knowledge of the onset in the energy dimension, we can better pinpoint the core of illness.

Process of Disease

The manner in which a disease unfolds is known as the pathology. This includes structural and functional changes in anatomy and physiology. Three basic areas of examination, done routinely, explain the process in reference to Western standards: physical examination, laboratory examination, and X-ray examination. Information gathered from a medical laboratory, X-ray facility, physical observation, combined with data from the initial history and consultation, gives us an extended basis for interpretation.

In addition to X-rays, scans and scope-type instruments, a variety of laboratory tests are used to study medical concerns in anatomy, chemistry, microbiology, and psychology. Deviations from normal values signify a disorder. Blood samples have the potential to show major disease-related changes. Three types of cells are present in the blood stream with specific purposes:

(1) Red blood cells contain iron-based pigment called hemoglobin, which allows the transportation of oxygen from the lungs to the tissues. Lab tests count the red cells, study their shapes and sizes and calculate the quantity of hemoglobin present.

(2) White blood cells come in different shapes, sizes

and types. Most play a major part consuming and eliminating bacteria. In the presence of infection, they increase in number. Increases and decreases have diagnostic importance. Some produce antibodies to aid immunity.

(3) Platelets are small irregularly shaped cells. They act to coagulate (clot) blood and stop bleeding. Their numbers may increase or decrease in various conditions.

Blood chemistry assessments take place in another laboratory department on portions of blood without cells (serum). Elevations and decreases when compared to normal values, point to disease conditions.   Some body substances studied include calcium, cholesterol, glucose, potassium, protein, sodium, and uric acid.

A range of tests, from blood and urine to cerebral spinal fluid, expose abnormalities and infection. Using contaminated body fluid, a culture is grown on a media to identify the organism. Reactions to the placement of antibiotic discs on the culture will tell which one is most effective.

When other means cannot provide necessary information to make an accurate diagnosis, a biopsy is considered. Biopsy, a surgical procedure, lets us examine cellular pathology. On this level, we can grasp the disease in depth. To reduce tissue injury, doctors often choose a needle biopsy for organs. Bone marrow, liver and kidney biopsies are commonly performed.

Many years ago, I worked in a hospital laboratory where many tests were painstakingly done by hand, using microscopes and test tubes. Advancements now employ advanced instrumentation to rapidly and precisely process specimens.

Acupuncture, in contrast, understands the disease process by patient consultation and physical examination. Results from conventional laboratory and X-ray findings may add information to the Chinese medical assessment. But the most valuable direction for an acupuncturist is through Traditional Chinese Medicine. Parallels can be drawn between normal and abnormal energy physiology. This relates to conditions of energy circulation such as blockages and stagnancy in the flow, pathogenic influences from climatic changes, functions and malfunctions of Organs, adequate amounts of Qi, Channel connections and afflictions from prolonged negative emotions.

Qi Energy

To comprehend the workings of healthy and unhealthy energy, we must explore basic principles. Most importantly, Qi energy powers the entire body and has life-sustaining responsibilities. Organs contain working Qi. Blood partners with Qi to circulate throughout the body. Qi travels pathways within us and connects to Organs. For better energy awareness, as previously mentioned, a customary practice in Chinese medical literature capitalizes words that refer to the intricate presence of Qi. Thus we have Blood, Organ, Channel, Kidney, Liver, etc.

Disharmonies between the physical content of blood and its Qi will result in a number of disorders. When not normally energized, Blood can Stagnate, Congeal and form Blockages, which impede the transport of nutrients to damaged tissue. Degeneration regenerates with the right corrective revitalization. Injury brings on hurtful effects to both physical structure and Blood. Take for example a case of diabetic ulceration on the foot from trauma. To heal the condition, Qi must at first return to the foot, and then Blood with its healing elements follows the Qi.

A fundamental guide of Chinese medical physiology centers on the precept of Yin and Yang, which looks at everything in terms of connected opposites. Cold and Hot, Wet or Damp and Dry, Deficiency and Excess, illustrate some Yin-Yang examples. Qi, by the way, is Yang and Blood is Yin. If a weakened patient suffers from a dry persistent cough, very likely a Lung Yin Deficiency—confirmed by tongue and pulse exams—will be recognized. Excess Damp Toxic Heat depicts a predominantly Yang condition and could furnish support for a bacterial infection.

Yin-Yang paired Organs attached in a rotating cycle by a network of Channels (energy pathways), inform us where the dysfunctional Qi exists. One Organ provides for or regulates another. Channels project from an Organ, similar to arteries carrying blood from the heart. Energy Organ sources and the uninterrupted flow of Qi, must remain in good working order to maintain a healthy physical body. Pathogenic elements such as detrimental invasions from the outside environment, injuries, insect and animal bites, poor diet, and prolonged negative emotions will disrupt the smooth spread and vital activities of Qi.

Negative emotions have significance for both Chinese and Western medicine. To the Chinese, when prolonged, they prove to be causative factors for disease. This goes the other way too. Physical ills will have detrimental psychological outcomes. Western medicine leans more toward the occurrence of the physical ailment causing mental problems.

Diagnosis of Disease

With emphasis on disorders in anatomy, chemistry, microbiology, and psychology, our medicine frequently took Greek and Latin words and syllables to formulate diagnostic terms. At times, the name of the discoverer labeled the ailment and once in awhile we find geographic reference. Colitis defines inflammation of the colon. Maurice Raynaud noticed color changes on the extremities from vascular disturbance, now known as Raynaud's Disease. Diabetes means passing through in Greek and one aspect is increased urination. Lyme Disease is a type of arthritis caused by a deer tick's infectious bite. It was first recognized as a distinct entity from a cluster of cases that occurred in Lyme, Connecticut. The word depression comes from the Latin meaning of pressing down.

Acupuncture frequently establishes a diagnosis through Qi energy Organ Syndromes or Patterns. A diagnosis in Western medicine may be a symptom in the Pattern. The Syndrome Deficient Kidney Yin could include hypertension, nephritis, constipation, and diabetes.

General Classifications

A general alphabetic comparison between Western medicine's disease classifications and Qi interpretations lays down parallel ways of thinking. These divisions mainly stress anatomical and chemical imperfections that correlate with energy faults. Comparable knowledge will improve medical standards.

Endocrine Glands form a system of hormonal secretions needed for reproduction, growth, and metabolism. The pituitary, thyroid, and adrenals represent some of the glands working together in the biochemical interactions. Acupuncture gives attention to related Organ and Channel energies. Adrenals sit on the Kidneys, so Kidney Qi reacts with them. The thyroid is situated along a particular neck Channel, through which thyroid function is influenced.

Gastrointestinal (GI) Disorders can occur from the esophagus to the rectum. Tissue changes (i.e., polyps), are often sources for discomfort and disorder. Infection, systemic disease, ingested toxin, obstruction, and psychological factors like a nervous stomach, merit consideration. In a similar way, Chinese medicine takes into account the entire digestive system, but in a functional Organ framework called The Triple Burner or Triple Warmer. The Upper Warmer contains the esophagus; the Middle Warmer, the Stomach and Spleen; the Lower Warmer, Liver and Intestines. Problems arise from negative feelings, pathogenic elements, and Stagnancy. These enter the GI tract. Stagnant circulation could foster tissue growths and Stagnant metabolism creates numerous digestive problems.

Geriatric Specialization (Geriatrics, Gerontology) is the study of the psychological and biological aspects of aging. Treating ailments associated with the elderly has importance in Chinese medicine. It recognizes an Inherited Qi, defined as Essence that stays with all humans throughout their lives. Aging takes place with the decline of this energy, which in the process, brings on certain illnesses like arthritic changes of the knees and lower back. Essence cannot be replaced but can be nourished and strengthened.

Gynecology and Obstetrics are two specialties dealing with female reproductive organs. They are often combined to form a specialty that evaluates and treats menstrual disorders, infertility, and prenatal symptoms, as well as delayed labor. Irregular structures and hormonal impairment may require drugs or surgery. But in Chinese medical terms, Blood-Qi Deficiencies or Excesses, or perhaps an abnormal, internal environment condition in the uterus, call for acupuncture or herbs.

Heart Conditions are numerous. Physical examination, electrocardiogram (ECG), stress tests, chest X-rays and, when necessary, echocardiography will provide diagnostic information.

Arteriosclerosis, coronary artery, and mitral valve diseases are familiar maladies. In the presence of palpitations, shortness of breath or chest pain, there will be searches for obstructions, abnormal contraction of heart muscles or valve discrepancies. Chinese medicine evaluates Qi and Blood Deficiencies, Stagnancy, and Heat Excesses. The Heart has much to do with sleep, speech, and emotions.

Hematology is the study of blood. Through laboratory exams, components of blood are counted, measured or analyzed. Routinely performed is blood typing for compatible transfusions. As a Qi-Blood Yin-Yang association, Qi directs and normalizes Blood. Anemia, white cell defects, and bleeding disorders are major diseases often helped by acupuncture.

Immunology explains the body's defenses through the biochemistry of antibodies and actions of certain white blood cells that consume pathogenic bacteria and toxins. In Chinese medicine, a weakened immunity often results in allergies. Disease prevention depends on defenses. A distinct energy known as Protective Qi surrounds the body and connects to the Lung and related Organs. A strong immune system to prevent allergies relies on this external complex.

Infections frequently have reference to the body part affected and the pathogenic organism. Bacterial meningitis describes infected meninges, which are membranes covering the spinal cord and brain. Indicated drug therapy attempts to do away with the bacterial evildoers. The toxic environment of the infection requires changes according to Chinese medicine. By restoring a healthy interior, the infection disperses. Acupuncture and herbs may do the job.

Liver and Gallbladder have a close working relationship in both Western and Chinese medicine. Western therapy targets jaundice, cirrhosis, hepatitis, tumors, fat, and gallstones. Chinese understanding finds these diseases also linked to disharmonies in other Organ Qi Syndromes. Through another process of pathology, acupuncture grew aware of rising energy connections from the Liver to the head, especially to the eyes.

Lung Diseases involve airway obstruction, infections from various microorganisms, occupational gases and dusts, cigarette smoking, abscesses, and tumors. Chinese medicine says the responsibility to govern Qi, respiration, and of note, immunity, lies with the Lung. Disturbance, therefore, commonly causes debilitation. In addition, Yin-Yang imbalances, harmful invasions and Phlegm retention do their damage. Phlegm is a pathological factor sometimes used as part of a Syndrome's name, for example, Retention of Damp Phlegm in the Lung Syndrome.

Musculo-Skeletal Disorders mainly refer to different forms of arthritis. Differential diagnoses compare signs and symptoms in order to select the arthritic type. Physical examination, X-rays, and lab tests help in the evaluation. Practitioners of acupuncture, herbal medication, and Chinese massage therapy know that Kidney Qi controls bone. When deficient, as in Kidney Qi Deficiency Syndrome, arthritis very likely appears. Likewise, working through Kidney Qi treats the problem.

Nerves, the Spinal Cord and Brain all belong to the specialty of neurology. Assessment of many problems, done from reflex testing to magnetic resonance imaging (MRI), identifies damage to a nerve or area of the brain. Some problems treated include insomnia, sensory losses, tremors, plus head and spinal injuries. Acupuncture evaluates and treats nervous system afflictions through penetrating energy and along associated Channels. Scalp acupuncture often proves helpful.

Nutrition and Malnutrition in Western science means either

sufficient or deficient nutrients in vitamins, minerals, and protein. Chinese medicine looks at therapeutic values in various foods, but also the harm from an abundant cold, rich, spicy, and greasy diet. Organ energies most often injured are Spleen Qi and Stomach Qi.

Skin Lesions, Inflammation and Infections are easily seen for examination. Diagnosis may not be so easy. While a medical student, I was told that a good book on dermatology must have many pictures, which is helpful in recognizing and treating patterns of lesions, dermatitis, infections, and eruptions. Again Chinese routines incorporate tongue and pulse exams to find causes. These develop from pathogenic wind or toxic invasions and pathogenic internal elements that surface. By consultation one also learns too of prolonged negative emotions. Everything is taken into account. The status of Qi-Blood skin circulation also needs evaluation.

Tumors require microscopic cellular examination. Whether localized or spreading (metastasis), Western medicine is aware of carcinogens, but admits to uncertainties in etiology. Chinese medicine interprets cancerous or benign growths with pathology of Stagnation, Toxic Heat, Turbid Dampness, and weak Organ function.

Urinary Problems continue to increase with growing needs for dialysis. Kidney disease, stones, injury and diabetes cause or contribute to the disorders. Genital problems are related. Chinese medicine places a comprehensive power of operations on Kidney Qi, the foundation of all body activity. It stores the vital Essence, governs growth and reproduction, and controls urinary and sexual energy.

Treatment of Disease

As different as Western and Chinese medicine may appear, they both plan their treatments on diagnostic findings. In cases of tumor formation, surgery removes the impaired cells and tissues. Radiation therapy and chemotherapy aim to destroy cancerous growths. In China most cancers are treated with acupuncture and herbs, but Western diagnostic methods have become widely used. Chinese treatment activates Stagnation, clears Toxins, regulates Organs and strengthens Immunity.

Physicians regard themselves in specialties as either surgical or medical. Of course, a surgical complication of infection may require the input of a medical infectious disease specialist. Another position divides health fields into physical or mental. Chinese therapies separate applied tactile skills, acupuncture and massage therapy, from herbal prescriptions. Like surgery to drugs, in essence, two separate health professions work with the same basic principles in all their subspecialties across the board. However, as emphasized previously, the physical and mental are not divided.

Chapter 4
My Way to a Healthy Life

Flow Out the Energy

As I studied Chinese Medicine for almost four decades, secrets of health kept surfacing. These I would like to share with you. However, please realize that not all routines apply to everyone. It's a matter of individual comfort when one accepts and uses a method. You must like what you are doing. Personally, I find benefit in combinations, which include Western holistic medicine.

Not too long ago, a Master of Qigong by the name of Duan Zhi Liang was invited to the United States to teach his style of a deep-breathing, energy-vitalizing exercise. Called Qigong, this method of healing has been proven to correct disease, including high blood pressure and cancer. Master Duan resides in Beijing, as the only surviving employee of the last Ch'ing Dynasty emperor who lived in the Forbidden City. Like his father and grandfather, he served as a doctor and bodyguard. Note that in China, a person's family name precedes the given name. Also the title Master denotes authority in a certain field, with years of experience.

Acupuncture, herbs, moxa, and massage therapy, are part of Master Duan's medical regimen for patients. To see him spar in martial arts with an upper hand, during good-natured sessions with men almost eighty years his junior, amazed me. A demonstration was performed, showing how energy from his palm was transferred and detected on a piece of cloth. Members of the audience, myself included, felt vibrancy as we grasped the material. I cannot give a total explanation of the experience. This powerful force, which the audience felt, effected strong healing while doing massage. In the middle of the evening, he administered therapeutic massage to volunteers aided by his young-looking wife. Then afterwards for entertainment, he jumped on a table and sang Chinese opera.

I asked a friend who spoke better Chinese than I, if she would find out his secret for longevity, limitless energy, and an extremely wholesome condition. Now in his nineties, did he use a special herb or acupuncture technique or a type of massage? After a few days, she replied to me that his secret was in Qigong. Ever since, I have adopted the Qigong motions as a morning ritual.

Since Chinese antiquity, many forms of Qigong have developed. It remains the basis of Tai Chi Chuan or Tai Ji, which consists of a series of structured exercises. Yoga brings about similar results. In addition, martial warriors fight using the same principles. Any physical movements can be converted to deep-breathing, energy-flowing actions. On observation, I noticed how Master Duan walked in a dynamic harmony as if he was floating.

I do not run or jog, but I enjoy long walks. Feeling and directing circulation through my legs and arms, while taking and absorbing breaths of air, permits me to do the Qigong walk. Not exhausting, but rather invigorating, it becomes a healthful activity.

People may question the value of incorporating Chinese health practices into daily life. Documentation of benefits over the centuries, to me serves as proof, even though it does not fit Western medicine's way of research and measurement by our standard instruments. Since Chinese medicine leans toward subjective results and I certainly feel the healthy responses, what do I have to lose? Every morning, masses of Chinese citizens follow leaders in exercise groups throughout the country. They find cures for disease and maintenance of well being. Is it a waste of time and effort? I think not.

Our Gifts from Nature

There was a man in China, a professor of herbs actually, who died in 1933. The following week, *Time Magazine* ran a feature on Monday, May 15, 1933, with an amazing piece of information, namely that he was born in 1677. That's right, Professor Li Chung Yun (spelled also Li Ch'ing Yuen) lived 256 years, confirmed by authorized records at Chengdu University where he taught. It does not seem possible for someone to live a biblical example of old age in the twentieth century. The question remains, can we find the secret to his longevity? Facts are known about Professor Li, but not everything.

Many acknowledge his extensive understanding of herbs. In his youth, he and three teachers went on an educational journey through China and other South Asian territories. They learned at length the applications of medicinal plants. He then practiced as an herbalist and gathered and sold his own plant products. Later he taught herbal medicine in a Szechwan province university. We know what he taught, as well as his advice for a long life. For instance,

47

he said keep a quiet Heart, which suggests a calm emotion without stress. Sit also like a tortoise (possibly a state of relaxation), but walk briskly, like a pigeon. This may mean the Qigong walk, since he performed Qigong exercises. Fourthly, sleep like a dog sleeps soundly.

Specifics on Professor Li's choices of medicine fall into a category of strength-induced or tonic herbs. If you have interest in taking these substances, it would be best to seek the guidance of an authoritative practitioner in the field. Some are ingested separately and some in combination. On top we find Ho Shou Wu or Polygonum multiflorum in Latin. This enhances Blood, Qi and hair growth. Professor Li mixed it with a deer antler extract. Since then, deer tail extract has shown benefits as well. Other herbs include ginseng and Lycii berries.

A word of caution: tonic herbs should not be taken during an acute illness, for instance a head Cold. Otherwise, the herbs will prolong the condition like obnoxious visiting relatives who will not leave your home. So clear the problem first with acupuncture or other indicated Chinese medicine. Then resume the tonic supplement.

Herbal teas and tablets have become a part of my lifestyle. To maintain a wholesome existence and correct ailments, I use herbs and treat myself with acupuncture. I must also mention that I employ these methods for disease prevention. In my office I have an herbal pharmacy, from which I supplement acupuncture treatments. Patients often refill their herbal prescription for maintenance care, sometimes for long periods.

A Closer Look at Japan

For more than a thousand years, adaptations of Chinese medicine have found a place in Japan. Modifications and refinements came about using gentler stimulation. Their inventiveness gave us a needle-cylinder method of insertion and waterproof, tiny needle attachments to the skin. In recent times an advanced application of Chinese-origin scalp acupuncture developed.

Their use of ignited moxa, with innovations, exceeds that in China. Seemingly as old as needles, the Chinese term for acupuncture—mentioned earlier—translates as needle-burn. It grows in many areas around the globe including America. But we consider the silvery-leaf plant a weed, called mugwort. Moxa is the Japanese name for mugwort.

A Japanese group of people routinely administers moxa heat to an acupuncture point on both legs, referred to by the name "walk three miles" or Stomach 36. Historically in China, the point was stimulated when hikers became tired and needed renewed endurance. It also supports a major source of immunity. Those who warm the region regularly live a long healthy life, over one hundred years. This self-help procedure may or may not have merit, but I feel a little extra time and effort in a day could possibly yield great health benefits. So now almost every morning after my Qigong exercises, I light up a moxa stick and heat my Stomach 36. Courses of study, presented by the Center for Chinese Medicine in Los Angeles, of which I was a member, explained and demonstrated this application.

Through the years, I discovered additional acupuncture points that respond well to moxa. Located on the legs, feet, abdomen and back, they enhance immunity and the inherited energy. After the therapy, I always experience an enhanced breath. Easier and safer to receive from another, until I mastered the skill for self-application, I burned myself several times. Professionally, I commonly use moxa in the office to supplement acupuncture. In China and elsewhere, mineral plate infrared heat lamps frequently serve as a substitute for the burning herb. China manufactures these lamps.

Living with the Change of Seasons

Many ancient Chinese principles of health actually developed from observing seasonal changes. Disease-producing elements that afflict the body relate to each part of the yearly cycle. To prevent sickness, one must understand the changing environment and how it affects us. Traditional Chinese Medicine recommends balancing the Yin and Yang (Cold and Hot) of weather by guarding against potential harm. The profound concept of Yin and Yang is the basis of diagnosis and treatment as well as prevention.

You can find advice to keep healthy through the seasons in the oldest book of medicine. Written over two thousand years ago, it's called the *Yellow Emperor's Classic of Medicine*. Let's go around the calendar, with the means and knowledge to stay well.

In autumn, do not overheat yourself with heavy clothing. Expose yourself to cooler air as comfortably as you can. However, on windy days, always protect the back of your head and neck. The ideal article of clothing to accomplish this is the scarf. A turtleneck serves the same purpose. Living in New England, I usually do not turn on the heat in my house until after Thanksgiving. Early to bed and early to rise, so you can subject yourself to the morning coolness. The goal in the months of fall aims to toughen your outer energy and close the pores of your skin, in preparation of the oncoming winter. I have noticed every year that I comfortably enjoy the colder months with this type of regimen.

When winter arrives, it is time to protect yourself. Early to bed, but late to rise. If you're able, sleep a little more in the morning with heat turned up. Dress snugly and remember the scarf. There are two acupuncture points behind the head at the base of the scalp. Named Pools of Wind, because Wind enters this region generally with—depending on the time of year—Cold, Damp or Heat. Disease-making elements invade and can penetrate deeply to cause other serious problems. Acupuncture therapy for colds, bronchitis and stomach virus, will needle Pools of Wind to clear the invasion and subsequent complications.

We must focus on prevention. The scarf should cover the base of the scalp to hamper the invasion, but the nose and mouth also become susceptible during cold, windy wintry days. As needed, wrap your scarf around the nose and mouth. If you take a walk in the blustery, bitter cold, without the prescribed head protection, you may later experience coughing, sneezing, and a runny nose. Then try it with the defensive covering and you will minimize symptoms.

With patience and endurance, finally comes spring, which we joyously welcome. Daylight lengthens, as weather grows warmer. We see nature's rebirth. It's a time to bed down early and wake early to seize some heat from the morning sunrise. Nevertheless, be cautious. Even though the out-of-doors feels warm, pockets of cold winter still remain. So, on a windy day, wear a sweater or jacket, collar turned up in back to defend against invasion.

In the spring of certain years, outbreaks of meningitis occur on college campuses. The disorder defines an inflammation, and an infection, of the meninges, which are membranes that cover the brain and spinal cord. It is partially a mystery as to why this happens. Chinese medicine offers some insight. The weather becomes warmer and brings forth the desire in men to remove their shirts, while they are outside. They are now more vulnerable to get the disease without the shielding at the back of the head and neck.

And now summer, the season of Yang heat arrives, and replaces the Yin cold. Stay up late and arise early. Wear fewer clothes and drink a lot of tea. No matter how hot, tea still has its Yin quality.

As a warning, take in the benefits of warmth without the excess of Summer Heat. The hot condition presents itself as a disease entity with sweating, dryness, and headaches leading toward emotional upset. Benjamin Franklin said early to bed and early to rise makes a man healthy, wealthy, and wise. Chinese medicine says that this pattern only applies in spring and fall. You should attempt to live in harmony with external conditions and adjust to the changes. For purposes of health, specific sleep patterns and wardrobes apply to individual seasons.

Seasonal conditions in northern China, where these health principles were formulated, reflect those of the northern United States. Tropical areas would follow different standards.

Skills of Massage Therapy

Benefits of massage therapy have gained increasing recognition in recent years. Many regard it as an adjunct luxury to mainstream medicine. Be that as it may, in China, massage is part of mainstream medicine, a medical specialty, performed by physicians. Large hospital clinics devote themselves to this hands-on application, used for centuries and called Tui Na or An Mo.

A segment of my hospital training took place in these clinics. I observed and participated in the rehabilitation of serious disabling problems. Each procedure has a Chinese name for an exact manipulation. There are even subspecialties. I spent time with a physician who treated childhood diseases. While the child sat on the mother's lap or was held by the mother, manual circular or linear pressures were put to use. Effective results frequently appeared immediately.

When my young grandson suffered from an uncomfortable stagnation problem of digestion, I treated him with Chinese pediatric massage. He felt so much relief that he gave me the plastic instruments from his little doctor kit.

I believe every type of therapeutic adjustment or massage provides benefits to prevent and treat ailments. My experience with Swedish technique, Japanese shiatsu, and Chinese application has proven to be beneficial. Some routines in China's clinics resemble chiropractic. In America, I have found chiropractic very helpful. Rolfing, another valuable therapy, works on connective tissue, to balance the whole body. I have personally gained better postural alignment.

For health maintenance, I receive massage therapy on a weekly basis. For awhile, I suffered from carpal tunnel syndrome, which was corrected by my massage therapist. Beyond giving relief to physical problems, emotional stress decreases during the session. It's a perfect time to unwind and enter a meditative state.

Balance Yang Activity with Yin Rest

During my fifteen-year association and preceptorship with Dr. Wan from Beijing, I noticed that after lunch he would rest on a treatment table. This was after a busy morning and before a busy afternoon. When I lived and trained in the Chinese hospital in Guangzhou, I observed the same thing. Following lunch, doctors and nurses hopped up on treatment tables for a midday siesta, lasting about a half-hour. The clinic shut down at this period. I adopted the practice and was refreshed for an active afternoon.

In the East, different forms of meditation practices are quite common. As a way for self-help, both inactivity and activity need equalizing. The Chinese philosophy of Yin and Yang must be used. Sit like a tortoise and walk like a pigeon.

These meditative intervals serve as a means of preventive

medicine. Since prolonged negative emotions cause a number of diseases, and calmness reduces mental disturbance, it also reduces illness. Of course, all mental unrest receives help. This also has an influence on people in good shape, to maintain and strengthen their soundness of mind and body. Health habits of the healthy will keep them healthy.

Eat For Good Health

Chinese culture puts herbs and food in one category. They're both prepared for health. In the traditional Chinese hospital, one finds herbal and dietary recommendations at the clinic of Internal Medicine. The difference between these products occurs in the amounts. Small quantities of herbs are used to produce change, and food combinations are indicated for a healthy life. When my associate Dr. Wan and his wife used to invite me to their home for dinner, they explained the medicinal value in everything served.

Rice is Nice

About 80% of Chinese meals consist of white rice, not brown but white, which is husked of its nutrients. The point of this preparation lies in the purpose rice has in the diet. Foods fall into categories by degrees of Yin and Yang. No matter how hot or cold a food substance, an intrinsic Yin or Yang quality remains. Celery, for example, stays Yin in spite of excessive boiling. Garlic is Yang even if frozen. Chinese principles recommend diversity of food intake, but not too many rich and fatty meals. Rice acts as the great Yin-Yang neutralizer at dinner, lunch, and breakfast. Japan also dines with white rice. I feel that rice noodles have a similar benefit.

My Cup of Tea

China's eating habits lean toward cooked food, and for good reason. When cooked, it already comes partially digested and made easier to digest completely. Additionally, too much Cold in the stomach will cause digestive disorders. Hot soups are common fare, sometimes in the middle of a meal. However, more than anything else, sipping from a cup of hot tea throughout the day, keeps the stomach warm. Often older Chinese sip only boiled water, but tea ingredients furnish medicinal particles and taste.

While working in the Chinese hospital, and through each day, I saw red thermos type containers with a handle on the side. These were filled with hot water and distributed with tea bags, to the clinics, patients' bedsides and to my private room once in the morning and once at night. Doctors, nurses, and patients all had their tea. In retrospect, I remember Dr. Wan as he brewed and drank tea between treatments of patients. His tea mug consisted of a decorative porcelain vessel and a colorful porcelain cover that kept the tea warm. I was so impressed by the ingenuity of this functional object of art that a friend gave me one for a present.

Thousand-years-old discoveries and customs, to promote health in China, are being followed by more recent Western type scientific exploration. This research uses chemical analyses and clinical studies. The popular green tea has been shown to reduce cholesterol, heart disease, stroke, and prevent certain cancers. It acts as an antioxidant and detoxifies the liver. Western acceptance of tea is growing, based on Western types of studies. Black tea has also been shown to have beneficial effects. Nevertheless, I have embraced green tea as a favorite beverage.

Cook For the Territory and Climate

Patrons of Chinese restaurants know quite well that food dishes vary from province to province, from spicy Szechwan and Hunan to the blander Cantonese. Recipes use Yin and Yang ingredients accordingly. Wet, swampy areas need drying spices and southern sultry climates crave balance with Yin edibles. Duck is very Yang, therefore the famous Peking Duck fits the menu for the colder, northern Beijing area.

I have a friend who owns and operates a local Chinese establishment. He tells me that ingredients change with the seasons. Knowledge in traditional cooking with Yin-Yang standards enables him to prepare food appropriate for the time of year. He also grows Chinese vegetables in his garden for use in his restaurant.

A Healthy Combination from East and West

Many findings and contributions for healthy eating are made in the United States. I try to take the best from both worlds. In 1976, Dr. Benjamin Frank authored a very popular book entitled *Dr. Frank's No-Aging Diet*. Unfortunately it is no longer in print. The book discusses nucleic acids in the forms of DNA and RNA found in food. The message of the book is that this in turn enhances the DNA and RNA in our bodies, keeping us younger and healthier. After intense research, it was revealed that certain food categories contain higher and lower amounts of nucleic acids.

The greatest content of nucleic acids is found in canned sardines. Salmon, mackerel and other types of fresh fish supply good amounts too. Beans and peas are contributors, especially pinto beans, lentils, garbanzo beans, black-eyed peas, small white beans, and large lima beans. Other sources include nuts, spinach, oatmeal, wheat germ, asparagus, mushrooms, radishes, and onions. A special function of beets activates us to produce our own individual nucleic acids. Meat products of note include beef liver and dark meat from chicken.

In subsequent decades, a major discovery featured omega-3 fatty acids. Its ingestion promotes improved function of the brain, cardiovascular and immune systems, and lowers cholesterol. Omega-3 fatty acids of course are found in one of the same places as nucleic acids, namely in saltwater fish: sardines, salmon, mackerel and tuna. Observe how sardines supply both omega-3 fatty acids and nucleic acids.

Many attribute the wholesome longevity of the Japanese to their large consumption of fish. Some eat fish three times a day. I truly enjoy a lunch or dinner of raw fish starting with miso soup, which has a soybean fermented base. Rather than sushi, I prefer sashimi that comes without the rolled rice. However, a side bowl of rice and refills of green tea give me an inner glow of energy.

The Chinese eat fish whole and separately, instead of chopped in vegetables. Being from the saltwater sea, fish aids the far reaches of Kidney energy that manages the skeletal system. A food therapy to relieve arthritis derives from the eating of fish and rice. However, in spite of all this, I have met older, healthy people who rarely consume fish.

A Few Personal Favorites

Everyone seems to have eating related habits, either for health or just to satisfy cravings. Vitamin supplements provide nutrition, particularly when lacking in one's daily diet. I also take supplements, but in the form of minerals. On the premise that our farming soils have been depleted of numerous minerals, replacements are necessary. Mixed in water, during the day I drink a liquid supplement, which includes trace minerals.

Traditional Chinese cuisine incorporates no dairy products (including yogurt), which is commonplace in neighboring India. Yogurt contains cultures of desirable bacteria that support the intestinal flora. I find it a good digestive aid.

An old continual practice in Western civilization concerns fasting. I have not come across this food abstinence custom in China, where the belief persists, to replenish the body with energy every day. Developed in United States, one type of cleansing fast consists of ingesting only fluids from vegan sources: vegetable broth, vegetable juice, fruit juice, but no animal protein. Soon the body starts eating its own protein, consuming the bad stuff first, such as tumors. Obviously, it is an anti-cancer process, yet done for prevention. A side benefit reduces some fat and weight. I do the fast during a few selected weeks of the year, feeling very detoxified afterwards.

I like to combine self-help activities while adhering to a regular schedule. I begin most days with the longevity herb Ho Shou Wu, then Qigong exercises. Self-application of moxa coincides with sipping a deer extract solution. Before and after moxa, I do some eye exercises based on the Bates Method, which maintains and improves vision. I run my sight along the black border of a board, also focusing back and forth at a near object and then at a distant object. Palming the eyes, cupping the palms over both eye areas, has a powerful effect. The healing energy given off from the hand penetrates deeply. Next come herbal tea and breakfast.

Much of my life has been a search of ways to stay healthy while aging. Along the way, I add and subtract to that which I find most suitable, helpful, and available. In the early 1970s when I pursued studies related to acupuncture, I was introduced to Foot

Reflexology. The foot actually works as a micro-acupuncture system and connects to the entire body. By methods to find and release crystal accumulations, the reflexologist can evaluate and treat all disorders. Upon completion of the course by Dwight Byers, followed by certification, I experienced vast benefits from this method.

Every field of health care has much to offer. My preferences move toward natural ways to help heal and maintain the body. I do a self-evaluation by taking my own pulses and examining my tongue and facial complexion. Treatment also follows any discomfort found during self-assessment. Acupuncture, herbs, therapeutic diet or massage therapy restore a condition of well being. Never have I undergone a skin-incision surgery other than a circumcision at eight days old—I had no choice. Never have I taken a sick day from work. Even now at Medicare age, I have not purchased any Medicare supplemental plans. I signed up for Plan A (hospitalization); why not? It's free.

Respect Your Medical Choices

As already stated, best to seek professional guidance if you care to adopt any of the practices discussed, to your lifestyle. There is much to choose from. Advice by holistic practitioners authoritative in their fields may prevent mishaps. The same holds true for conventional medicine. Both approaches may call for second opinions. If avoidable, do not take random chances.

I respect peoples' medical choices, though different they may be. Our present medical crisis of lack of care for much of the population requires financial remedy. There are two parts to the situation. Firstly, much of the conventional care provided by insurance requires premiums unaffordable for many. And secondly, other, less costly

59

methods that remain uncovered, could possibly correct the sickness if used. The solution can be found in Chinese medicine

Traditional Chinese Medicine with consultation, pulse and tongue examination, and palpitation for tenderness, provides a wealth of diagnostic information. Without sophisticated equipment required for evaluation, fees stay at a minimum. Acupuncture needles and related medical supplies also remain relatively inexpensive. A session consisting of consultation, evaluation and treatment usually—but not always—has a favorable outcome. Reinforcements and maintenance may be necessary as levels of correction are achieved. Herbal medication also proves effective at reasonable prices.

Acupuncture and herbs treat a wide range of ailments, in adults and children. Based on thousands of years of successful application, Chinese medicine offers options for healthcare. In-depth studies of usage, consultations with acupuncturists and herbalists may reveal the direction for an improved healthcare system. Improvement will evolve with better results and cost containment.

Western and Eastern medicine need not be competitive, where one attempts to replace the other. Instead, they should coexist for the sake of the patient. Then we will arrive at better solutions for healthcare issues.

Chapter 5
Diseases According to Chinese Medicine

In the Chinese Hospital, after the patient examination, my teachers taught me diagnoses (i.e., Excess Cold in Lung, Damp Heat in Liver, Deficient Spleen Qi or perhaps Deficient Kidney Yin). These are actually syndromes or patterns arrived at by consultation and examination of the pulse and tongue—no X-ray studies, no scans, and no lab tests. Performed for thousands of years, the same procedures today prove effective and inexpensive.

Chinese and Western medicine look at disease in different ways. Conventional Western medical thinking focuses on cause and effect. Remove the cause and cure the illness. Bacterial infections respond to eliminating the bacteria with antibiotics. If a tumor is present, remove it surgically. Depression may require medication or psychotherapy to alleviate the negative emotion.

Principles of acupuncture require us to balance the imbalances. If too Hot, you cool it down, likewise, you increase the warmth if too Cold. Disharmonies between Dryness and Moisture need regulating

61

with the goal of harmonizing the Yin and Yang. Yin defines Cold and Damp; Yang defines Hot and Dry. Other serious pathology takes place in the form of Stasis of Qi and Blood, which calls for activation.

The internal environment that supports a bacterial infection involves Damp Heat or Yang in Yin. Treatment involves eliminating the pathogenic conditions within the body. Tumors can result from Toxic Stagnant Heat, which demands expulsion. Acupuncture and herbs accomplish these tasks. Furthermore, treatment strengthens immunity to help reverse the disease process, associated symptoms then decline.

Mental and Physical

When Western medicine looks for abnormal functioning in structure and body chemistry, acupuncture evaluates Qi energy dysfunction. The problem could happen in circulation where Qi and Blood flow together, or within Organ energy itself. Organs supply Qi, which moves through everything physical. One affects the other; Qi acts on body parts and body parts act on Qi.

Mental health also deals with invisible forces. Not only do prolonged negative emotions cause disorders, but each type of emotion associates with Organ energy. All feelings involve the Heart, and when intense, the Pericardium. Both psychological and physical disturbances are helped with acupuncture. Therapy balances Organ Qi and the mind. More directly, needle insertions in the head and ear stimulate brain and psychological healing.

The mind, anatomy, and physiology were never separated in China, as in the Western World. Syndromes often have both mind and body symptoms. Mental conditions are evaluated with the same diagnostic routines of consultation, pulse, and tongue observations. Several acupuncture points can remedy psychological and physical ailments at the same time. So the cause and the outcome heal together.

Chinese Symptom - Western Diagnosis

Disease patterns classified by acupuncture contain signs and symptoms that commonly coincide with a Western diagnosis. The Chinese name, however, identifies the pathology established by principles of energy disruption. For example, a form of pain is called Blockage Pain, since pain results from blockage of Blood and Qi circulation. Relief of the pain occurs after the circulation frees the blocking obstacle in that particular part of the body.

Another example concerns stroke. Called Central Wind and often translated as Wind Stroke, the disease process begins with a rising internal force. It goes from the Liver up through the Heart to the Brain, like a volcano. Phlegm and Heat may complicate the problem. Western medicine's knowledge of cerebral hemorrhage or aneurysm that brings on a stroke, results from acupuncture's recognition of an ascending internal Wind. Obviously, the Wind afflicts the Brain, which leads to vascular problems. The patterns are Liver Wind Ascending or Phlegm Heat Agitating the Heart. Note that the concept of Phlegm refers to a substance found in a number of different body areas. It contributes to and complicates disorders.

Invasions

Aside from ongoing pessimistic attitudes as causative factors of disease, pathogenic invasions with Wind can do their harm. When at the outer skin surface, our Protective Qi tries to hold back the intrusion. Heat or a slight fever adds to the defenses. But if unsuccessful, the intruders enter structures below the skin and then into Organs. The deeper the elements go, the more serious the problem, which may even result in fatality. Acupuncture or herbs, or both, frequently can expel the penetration.

A milder form of stroke does not begin in the Liver, but from invading Wind. Only superficial Channels are directly involved, mainly in the head. Facial paralysis may appear with eye and mouth deviations. In comparison, Western medicine blames disturbed circulation of the brain—specifically the cerebrum—as the stroke culprit. It was given the name CVA, which stands for cerebrovascular accident. In the Chinese medical way of thinking, pathogenic Wind causes all manifested signs and symptoms.

Although the dominant sources of illnesses relate to emotional and invasive happenings, other causes can play a roll. These include poor diet, toxic contamination, insect and animal bites, and injuries. And we must not forget congenital disorders due to deficient inherited energy.

A good diet balances Yin and Yang without too much cold or uncooked food. Meals should agree with seasons and weather. Toxic conditions can result from ingested poison, insect and animal bites, things the Chinese knew about for centuries, particularly during epidemics. Toxins also bring forth complications in certain disorders such as infection and cancer. Injuries are understood in terms of disturbance in the flow of Qi and Blood. A birth defect requires evaluation to rehabilitate Inherited Qi Deficiency.

Details of an ailment in regard to dysfunctional Organs and their signs and symptoms have a direct correlation with treatment. Patient examination immediately tells us to dispel Dampness, to clear Heat, to strengthen an Organ's Qi, to resolve Stagnation or to increase Yin or Yang.

Disease Descriptions

The following chapters list commonly known diseases, in alphabetical order, for easy reference. Each description deals with causes, pathology, and therapy. Comparisons between the Western and Chinese approaches reveal new insights into medical concepts for improved health care. Cross-references expand this comprehension. Also, I have interjected findings based on my forty years of patient care experience.

Chapter 6
Abscess to Autism

Abscess

Chinese and Western medicine recognize types of abscesses and the body parts so afflicted. Both medical fields are mindful of heat from inflammation and even a fever. Each recognizes the role of the immune system.

Western science understands a person's defenses of white blood cells that consume the causative organisms, the bacteria, which then expire to form pus (the abscess). Diagnostic measures attempt to identify the responsible organism by placing and growing a specimen on a suitable culture. Treatment commonly consists of draining the abscess and using antibiotics.

In comparison, the Chinese emphasize toxins, abnormal Heat, Damp Heat, Blood and Energy supply, and decreased immunity. Herbal and acupuncture treatment moves out the Heat and toxins, dries harmful Dampness, and replenishes healthy Blood-Qi circulation and, in addition, strengthens immunity Qi.

Bacteria will thrive in a weakened immune system with abnormal Damp Heat. Antibiotics may kill the culprits, but in Chinese medicine, a vitalized internal human condition will be very effective to correct the infection. Fresh Blood and Energy to the area helps repair damage.

In my experience, persistence of the Heat and Dampness may continue after antibiotic actions kill the pathogens. If you ever did a biology class experiment to grow a bacterial colony in a Petri dish, you know that heat and dampness are necessary. Of equal importance, abnormal Heat and Dampness in the human body encourages infection, which acupuncture and herbs abolish by the elimination of the Damp Heat.

Acne

An embarrassing pimple-blemish skin change, common during—but not limited to—the teenage years, appears mainly on the face and less frequently on the chest, shoulders, and upper back. Severity varies in depth, numbers and sizes of lesions.

Western medicine considers the causes to be hormonal changes. It also looks at hyperactive sebaceous, oily-substance, gland secretions in the top layer of skin. Another factor assumes the possible presence of bacteria. Therapies advise proper cleansing and choices of certain medication, which often include oral or topical antibiotics. Tetracycline has been used for many years.

Chinese treatments regulate Blood circulation to the skin, while cooling and removing toxins. Due to the resemblance, the condition is called "white thorns". It arises from five sources of Heat, alone or in combination, and exhibits related external signs in the skin. Heat can stem from (1) the Lung, (2) Stomach, (3) Blood, (4) toxins, and (5) Dampness with Blood Stagnation. Blood Heat has emotional links.

Treatment with acupuncture and herbs cools the Blood, eliminates Dampness, regulates Organ energy, drains toxins or strengthens emotions. Heat reduction remains a major focus of acne therapy. Instructions in diet and personal habits often supplement Chinese or Western medicine. My therapy usually combines acupuncture and herbs.

Addiction

By Western standards, dependence on substances like alcohol and drugs fall into two general categories of (1) psychological and, (2) physiological cravings. Behavioral studies show that certain addictive personality types often arise from a traumatic past. Though at first not very harmful, continued intake leads to dependence. It also leads to increases in attempts to reach the desired "high". Social acceptance, without abusing oneself and others, varies as a norm in Western and Asian cultures.

Therapy leans toward medication, counseling, and support groups. Keeping records of controlled substances, studying toxic damage to organs and documenting withdrawal symptoms, all add to the understanding of habitual (habit formed) behavior.

Acupuncture has gained international recognition in its methods to correct problems of addiction. Since Chinese medicine never separated the physical from the psychological and emotional, acupuncture applies to all areas. Evaluation may consider specific disturbed feelings; however, the main goal is acupuncture needle insertion that produces behavior modification.

(See also Alcohol, Drug, Addiction, Cigarette Addiction)

Addison's Disease
(See Cushing's Disease and Addison's Disease)

AIDS

Differences in attitudes of care by Western and Chinese medicine are found in the definitions of AIDS and HIV. The acronym AIDS is an abbreviation for Acquired Immune Deficiency Syndrome, manifested by various signs and symptoms such as periodic fever, swollen lymph nodes, headaches, rashes, diarrhea, weakness, weight loss, and tumors. Full-blown AIDS refers to a severe state of altered immunity. AIDS related complex (ARC) has milder signs and symptoms.

HIV stands for human immunodeficiency virus. The level of infection is marked by numbers of certain lymphocytes called T-cells. These white blood cells act to defend the body. Thus their quantity reflects one's state of immunity. A major goal of Western medicine aims to develop a vaccination for the AIDS virus and improve anti-viral drugs.

In contrast, Chinese medicine works on Organ and internal environment deficiencies. Symptoms with tongue and pulse examinations pinpoint troubled areas. Most often afflicted is the Kidney Yin Qi, whose imbalance leads to less Blood, Dryness of the skin and mouth, and low-grade fever. Additional distresses include disrupted Spleen Qi that agitates the gastrointestinal system, plus head ailments, respiratory inflammation, and emotional upset.

With the combination of Western medicine's diagnostic laboratory procedures and Chinese medicine's immune enhancing herbs and acupuncture, progress has been made. They work well together. However, the epidemic is far from being eliminated.

Alcohol Addiction

Frequent drinking of large amounts of an intoxicating beverage defines alcoholism. Uncertainties exist as to the true cause. Frustrating circumstances in life and loneliness illustrate two examples that may compel one to drink. Science understands alcohol absorption into the blood stream and subsequent organ damage. Among treatments, the organization Alcoholics Anonymous (AA) has been shown to be most helpful.

Acupuncture mainly treats alcohol, and other addictions, by needle stimulation to specific points on the ear. Called auricular therapy, the Chinese found that the ear is an extension of the brain and mirrors the entire body in miniature. This procedure offers many benefits for addictive disorders. Outside of China, countries have contributed to this technique, which includes the United States.

Usually done in combination, sometimes with needling elsewhere on the body, point selection is made based on an evaluation. Several ear points relax the patient, one serves as a precise addiction point, another strengthens emotions and others relate to Organ function. An important Organ energy concerns the Lung, which regulates the body's fluid passages. To continue the stimulation out of the office, some practitioners attach a small patch to an ear point that contains a tiny needle or ball bearing or a type of seed. These are very convenient, waterproof and easily removed.

(See Addiction)

Allergy

Western medicine defines allergies as hypersensitivity reactions to substances found in foods, drugs, perfumes, dusts, plants, pollens, metals, animals, molds and bacteria, to name a few. These chemical culprits that cause troublesome responses are called allergens. Yet, ill effects do not always take place and minimal happenings can go unnoticed.

The reaction occurs when injured cells release chemicals called histamines, causing bronchial asthma, hay fever, skin rashes, and itching. Hence treatment consists of antihistamines and possibly steroids. It also very much helps to avoid the related allergen. Allergists also recommend environmental controls.

Whereas Western medicine evaluates and treats allergies on levels of chemistry and microbiology, acupuncture probes and treats on the level of an energy syndrome, designated as Deficient Lung Qi. Chinese medicine recognizes a protective energy that arises from the Lung and covers the body, which opens at the nose and controls respiration. You can easily see why these external areas, prone to allergic reactions, have difficulties being distant from internal Lung Qi defensive influence. Weakness of this influence allows allergic reactions to occur.

To care for the Lung Deficient condition, acupuncture or herbs must strengthen the Lungs and the Protective Qi. An additional Organ function gives aid to the Lung. This relates to Spleen Qi, which clears excess Dampness anywhere in the body, including Phlegm congestion and a runny nose. With overall correction of Lung dysfunction, acupuncture then attends to individual symptoms such as sinus and nasal congestion, cough, watery eyes, and skin eruptions.

A specific disorder merits extra attention. Called nose discharge by the Chinese and allergic rhinitis by Western medicine, it occurs when the mucous membrane lining reacts to an allergen. This

71

uncomfortable chronic condition is sometimes diagnosed as hay fever.

Acupuncturists believe differently. The source comes from either Deficient Lung Qi or one of four disease-producing atmospheric invasions. Each presents its own symptoms. Cold Wind results in a white discharge with obstructed nostrils, sneezing, headache, cough, chills, and fever. Heat Wind shows a yellow discharge with obstruction, fever, cough, and thirst. Dry Heat produces nasal Dryness and obstruction, slight yellow discharge, bitter taste, and Dry throat. Damp Heat exhibits an excessive, thick pungent discharge, also nasal blockage, and heaviness in the head with discomfort and bitter taste.

Both evaluations are correct, depending on whether one diagnoses through anatomy and biochemistry or by energy and invading forces. However, acupuncture does have the advantage of directly treating the problem in Channels around the nose.

Amenorrhea

Amenorrhea defines a lack of the menstrual period, either never to have occurred beyond age eighteen or stopped after having active monthly flow. The former is called primary; the latter, secondary. Western medicine assesses dysfunction in reproductive organs, glands and their hormones. At times, an amenorrhea syndrome shows up after complications of an injurious curettage procedure, possibly due to infection. Other causes deal with abnormal structure, systemic diseases, and psychological stresses. Assessments rely on studies of anatomy, biochemistry, microbiology, or psychology. Treatments with medication, surgical repair, or counseling are used as indicated.

Acupuncture makes a diagnosis in terms of energy Organs and

Channels, and energized Blood. There are two general amenorrhea conditions, Stagnant Blood and Deficient Blood. To understand the energy of Stagnation, we must first understand the energy of menstrual physiology. We are talking here more in terms of energy than structure.

The Liver has the responsibility to evenly spread circulation. It also carries out the function of storing uterine Blood, which becomes transported to the uterus through two connecting Channels. Basically, Stagnant Liver Qi remains the source for the disorder, and the reason for Liver Stagnation is prolonged negative emotions like depression. There is a parallel in Western medicine's diagnosis of psychological stress. We have yet another contributing cause.

This stems from an internal Cold condition. Acupuncture needling and herbal remedies adjust Liver Qi and regulate uterine Blood to correct the trouble.

Deficient Blood presents a different course. Due to prolonged sickness or many exhausting pregnancies, depleted Kidney Qi weakens activities of the womb. In addition, reduced menstrual flow reflects loss of Spleen Qi that manufactures Blood. On occasion, Heavy Dampness (Phlegm) blocks and decreases Blood. Signs and symptoms of weakness accompany this illness in the form of loss of appetite, dryness, sallow complexion, and dizziness. Treatment centers on shaping up the Kidney Qi, which governs reproductive Organs, and improvements to Spleen Qi, and menstrual energy Channels.

Anemia

Both Western and Chinese medicine agree that anemia is more of a symptom than a diagnosis. An underlying disease or syndrome may cause an anemic condition, identified by reduced numbers of red blood cells or hemoglobin. Acupuncturists evaluate by physical examination such as Cold limbs, changes in the body, coating of the tongue, and failings in the pulse.

Western classifications list many different types of anemia. One occurs from excessive bleeding, others from iron deficiency, kidney or thyroid disorders, vitamin deficiency, destruction or defects of the red blood cell, and disorders of hemoglobin formation. Treatments consist of blood transfusions when indicated, and vitamin and mineral (iron) replacements, while identifying and correcting the underlying disease.

Acupuncture recognizes the Spleen in the production and management of Blood, also the holder of Blood in vessels to prevent bleeding. In Blood making, an additional Organ includes the Heart. Its energy governs Blood, Blood Vessels, and Pulses. The third Organ of the Blood administration team is the Liver, which stores Blood. When anemia appears, acupuncturists consider and treat various "Deficiency" Syndromes of the Spleen, Heart, and Liver.

Angina Pectoris

Characterized by chest pain and pressure, Western medicine views the cause as deficient oxygen to the muscle layers of the heart wall called myocardium. Diagnostic details are often provided by physical examination, ECG, imaging of blood vessels on an angiogram, and response to exercise (stress test). Obstruction of vessels supplying oxygen to the heart is the usual finding. In general, doctors focus on abnormalities of anatomy and biochemistry. The treatment plan might consist of therapy that restores sufficient oxygen, the under-tongue medication of nitroglycerin and, if needed, surgery.

Working in the dimension of energy, Chinese medicine interprets this serious Heart ailment as a painful obstruction of the chest due to Deficient Yang Activity or Stagnation of Qi and Blood. Phlegm-Dampness Stagnation could also obstruct Heart Qi, especially associated with obesity.

Based on acupuncture diagnosis, correction occurs by dispersing Stagnation or invigorating the Heart and the related Organ, the Kidney. Acupuncture, and herbal therapy with Western diagnostic methods (i.e., ECG), represent an excellent combination.

Anxiety
(See Emotions)

Anorexia

According to Western concepts of anorexia, behavioral and emotional disorders are expressed in denying oneself food. A distorted self-image and fear of weight gain mirror social standards of an acceptable appearance. Women may also experience amenorrhea. Binge eating (bulimia) followed by purging may also occur as a separate but related illness.

Acupuncture has a different take on the ailment. It is seen as Organ disturbances, mainly Spleen and Stomach. As a symptom, anorexia fits into a few syndromes. Bear in mind, however, the emotional causative factor, which in this case, is tied to worry.

Functions of the Spleen include managing the transportation of food and its transformation into Qi and Blood. Deficient Spleen Qi will reduce appetite—observe how production of Blood decreases resulting in amenorrhea. Stagnant Stomach Qi disrupts digestion. Deficient Stomach Yin appears where lubricating juices decrease and dryness interferes with food assimilation. Acupuncture can strengthen Spleen Qi, release Stomach Stagnancy, restore Stomach lubrication or Yin, and with improvement of emotions, can alleviate anorexia.

Appendicitis

When an appendage of the large intestine, named the appendix, becomes inflamed, the patient has appendicitis. If ruptured it could lead to peritonitis, a serious, possibly life-threatening infection of the peritoneum, the lining of the abdomen. Today's life-saving advances of removal of the appendix (appendectomy) and infection control are performed routinely. Other abdominal disorders can imitate symptoms of appendicitis, which physicians should keep in mind.

Acupuncture places this condition in a syndrome known as Stagnation of Blood and Heat in the Large Intestine or Intestinal Abscess. I have noticed that even after an appendectomy, painful symptoms continue from Stagnant Blood and Heat. Treatment, of course, consists of removing the Hot Stagnation. Frequently an acupuncture point at a distance from the diseased area becomes diagnostically and therapeutically effective. It so happens that a spot on the right leg grows tender in the presence of Abdominal Abscess, indicating urgency for acupuncture needling.

Appendicitis serves as an example in which Western medicine emphasizes anatomy and microbiology, and where acupuncture focuses on pathologic energy developments. One type of doctor treats the infection by surgical repair and infection control. The other type applies needle combinations to clear the Heat, regulate the colon and drain toxins.

Chinese herbal medication provides the same actions with compatibility and additional help. Furthermore, selected Western and Chinese methods can work together.

Arthritis

From a single definition of joint inflammation, broad categories of arthritis classifications have evolved. As a student, decades ago, I was taught that rheumatoid arthritis (RA) affected many joints with inflammation and eventual disability. Non-inflammatory arthritis of one or just a few localized joints was named osteoarthritis (OA). Then we have extra groups of traumatic arthritis, caused by injury; gouty arthritis, found with the metabolic disease of gout; and degenerative disorders such as osteoporosis. Reiter's syndrome consists of arthritis with eye and urinary tract inflammation. Psoriatic arthritis associates with the skin condition of psoriasis.

At present, extensive documentation covers connective tissue degeneration, nerve and spinal sources, a full range of infections, and disorders in body chemistry. Evaluation by physical examination is combined with laboratory testing, X-rays, scans and arthroscopic findings. Drug therapies and joint replacements offer relief. Also, many experience improvement from chiropractic services, massage therapy, and physical therapy.

Uncertainties as to the causes of arthritis (degenerative joint disease) have plagued medical minds for a long time, and continue to do so. Why should a joint become arthritic? Acupuncture may hold many of the answers, specifically in Deficient Kidney Essence and Painful Obstruction.

First, I'll give you a little background on the inherited energy that we all receive at birth. It comes from both parents and is then contained in the Kidney area throughout life. Though we cannot replace the inheritance, we can nourish and strengthen this energy referred to as our Essence. Among its functions are responsibilities for reproduction and growth from childhood, grasping Lung Qi as we breath and controlling the skeletal system—the arthritis connection. Gradual depletion of Essence over a lifetime results in the aging process and consequently, in arthritic degeneration, which initially takes place in the low back and knees. However, a localized fixed bone and joint degeneration from the Deficiency may appear as osteoarthritis.

Acquired energy complements inherited energy. It must be replaced every day, obtained by means of the food and herbs we eat, as well as liquids we drink, and air we breathe. Conversion of these substances and elements into energy basically occurs in our metabolism. We also transfer energy through the care we bestow on one another. The significant therapeutic principle here is that acquired energy nourishes our Essence.

The affliction of Painful Obstruction Syndrome may or may not include Kidney Essence Deficiency, though Weakness allows susceptibility. The pathologic process follows a sequence. At first, disease-producing weather elements invade and block Circulation. These distant, pathogenic conditions move and settle in joints, likely after a respiratory ailment such as the common cold.

The outcome results in a painful joint with signs and symptoms that relate to one or more of the invading elements listed as Wind, Cold, Dampness, and Heat.

Wind moves the pain to various joints. Cold restrains the discomfort but Heat gives rise to inflammation and swelling (Heat and Dampness). Actually, an incursion of Cold in certain circumstances can change to Heat. Dampness stays in the joint and brings about an uncomfortable sensation of heaviness. The longer the harmful intrusion remains, the worse it becomes. Combinations, such as Damp Heat, also aggravate the disorder. Western medicine sees the end result of these invasions, and will place them under the heading of rheumatoid arthritis.

Let us now review methods of treatment. The use of aspirin, whether inflammation is present or not, has long been a standard Western prescription, taken with precautions for stomach irritation. Steroids offer an anti-inflammatory outcome on a short-term and a long-term basis. Physician thinking is directed to body chemistry. But abnormal, decalcified structure often suggests the need for corrective surgery. At present, there are injections to replace joint fluid. Antibiotics assist in cases of infection, including Lyme Disease.

Chinese medicine concentrates on patient-experienced symptoms and the internal condition. Restoring normalcy comes about by manipulating the patient's energy. An obstruction is recognized as Wind, Cold, Heat, or Dampness and eliminated by the actions of needle insertions, herbal medication, or Chinese massage. Therapy strengthens Systemic Qi while circulation of Qi and Blood improves through Channels in and around the joint. Degeneration as a result of Essence deficiency requires attention to both Kidney and joint energy. In these situations, I will frequently apply an enhancing herbal heat known by its Japanese name of moxa. The herb is mugwort.

Acupuncture can supplement or possibly serve as an alternative to joint replacement surgery. People have requested acupuncture from me before and after a hip replacement, which significantly reduced the healing time. Then there was a woman in her forties who received a recommendation to replace her hip. Following a series of acupuncture treatments, her doctor said the operation was unnecessary. A man once came to me to prevent a knee corrective procedure. Acupuncture therapy eventually relieved his pain and fully restored knee flexibility.

Although Lyme Disease does not appear in traditional Chinese medical literature, I have had success using acupuncture principles. Infections fester in Damp and Heat (swelling and inflammation) with toxins. Treatment drains the toxic Heat and Dampness and restores healthy Blood and Qi circulation.

Asthma

Western medicine understands asthma as a bronchial disease, appropriately called bronchial asthma. It presents as constrictions in the bronchial tubes and blockages of airways.

Suddenly, breathing becomes difficult followed by wheezing, the whistling sounds. It is thought that allergic, infectious, or emotional factors stimulate reactions.

In Chinese medicine, the same symptoms of labored breathing and wheezing indeed associate with a diagnosis of an asthmatic condition. However, Phlegm obstruction remains the principle cause. Phlegm has a wider meaning in acupuncture than in Western medicine. In one set of illness-induced circumstances, the obstruction occupies the Lung; in another it has an affinity for Channels, joints, and various Organs.

In asthma, it could form due to a Cold invasion that activates the otherwise pathological state of hidden Phlegm. If the source stems from Heat Phlegm, you hear a louder and stronger form of wheezing. Organ energy responsible for preventing Phlegm accumulation takes into account Lung, Spleen, Stomach and Kidney. Their Deficiencies that impede the transformation and transportation of Body Fluids result in Phlegm. Pulse and tongue signs reveal causes and Organs involved. Nevertheless, the chief asthmatic offender points to the Spleen.

Compare anatomical dysfunction of bronchial tubes with Organ energy dysfunction in regard to therapeutic approaches. The mechanical-anatomy logic seeks to open the airways through a process called bronchodilation and to reduce inflammation. Testing and treating with dilators gain an important place to detect and clear blockages. Acute attacks require intravenous administration. Epinephrine and aminophylline relieve asthma attacks and have long been standard medications. Additional measures may warrant direct inhalation of oxygen and, in the presence of suspected infection, antibiotics. Also the use of steroids reduces inflammation.

Acupuncture works to correct the unhealthy condition in the body's internal environment. Asthma mainly pertains to the upper torso designated as the Upper Burner or Warmer. Three Burners known as the Upper Burner, Middle Burner, and Lower Burner function as parts of the energy Organ. The Upper Burner manages and takes in the Lung and Heart. Our attention now centers on the Lung factor. The Middle or Central Burner by the way, deals with digestion, and the Lower Burner with elimination.

Needling or herbal remedies, or both, apply directly to the different asthmatic syndromes. In a pattern of Excess Damp Phlegm Retention in the Lungs, the abundance must be removed through increased strength to the Lung and Spleen. When Cold Violates the Lungs, they need Warmth. Of course, a Wind Heat Invasion demands expulsion. Since Kidney Qi anchors the breath, enhancing Deficient Kidney Essence will greatly improve weak respiration.

Certain indicated points prove most effective. Needle stimulation above the breastbone known as the sternum, ventilates the Lung and augments elasticity of its tissues. A Spleen and Stomach meeting

81

point on the leg specifically clears Phlegm. Treatment to the upper back can aid a good result as well.

Asthma knows no age limits. A middle-aged woman with a long history of asthma-related problems came to see me. She had been under the care of a lung (pulmonary) specialist. Several acupuncture treatments restored normal breathing and cured the illness. Her pulmonary specialist then contacted me, as he was amazed to find that on clinical examination, the condition was resolved. He invited me to his office to discuss acupuncture and asthma. It was a friendly, productive meeting.

In an article I wrote for a holistic health magazine, I described how a twelve-year-old girl wheezed so loudly that she constantly disturbed her classroom. Since early childhood, her disorder had become worse and no one was able to help. A consultation revealed her emotional and Lung failings. Diagnosed as a Cold-Damp Lung Syndrome, I was able to correct her asthmatic condition and bring tranquillity to the teacher and students.

Autism

Autistic behavior begins early in life when the child has a self-centered focus with a wandering mind. This connects with a lack of social interaction and impaired speech development. Therapies to help the impairments are beneficial. Previously, brain injury was considered as a possible additional cause, but today's care emphasizes intellectual maturity.

How does acupuncture view this childhood dysfunction? Well, it offers knowledge of Deficient energy and much therapeutic assistance. A few different syndromes show their presence by symptoms. Energy deficiencies that became severe will affect the Kidney, Brain, and Emotional Heart where the Spirit resides.

Fostering Qi replacement, particularly the Heart's Spirit, enhances mental capacity.

Another pattern results from excess internal Heat, perhaps due to a high fever disease in infancy. Hyperactivity, irritability and a reddish complexion describe this state. The Heart also takes its share of Fire. Treatment endeavors to extinguish the excess. In opposition, a Cold disorder can emerge as a Kidney Essence or Qi Deficiency. Directed toward Kidney revitalization and warming energy with moxa, acupuncture aids the problem.

Emotional trauma or retained anger could also be at the core. Acupuncture needling applied to build up healthy feelings or draw out the negatives, may be useful. Children usually respond to minimal acupuncture insertions. Although degrees of correction may necessitate several sessions, it is worth the time for these children to improve.

Chapter 7
Backache to Drug Addiction

Backache

Ever experience pain in your back? Well, you're not alone. These types of problems have plagued sufferers throughout human history, as well as today. Many find relief and many do not. Without satisfactory treatment for everyone, we go on looking for causes and treatment. Western Medicine searches in terms of injury, poor posture, a spinal disk problem, fracture, and narrowing or stiffening of the spine. Pelvic infections or tumors also cause pain. The chiropractic profession has successfully cared for dislocations called subluxations.

In spite of the therapies offered by Western health professions, I still see a substantial number of back disorders. Reason being, Chinese Medicine interprets these ailments in a different way. Based on circulatory disturbances or Organ energy dysfunction, new perceptions of the problems can emerge to provide unique approaches for effective correction. Take for example, a low back sprain from heavy lifting and twisting. X-ray or scans can rule out or detect structural damage. Areas of pain correlate with anatomical knowledge of specific nerves and muscles. Acupuncture by contrast recognizes Channels in the region, in which flow energy and Blood. Trauma, unfortunately, will stagnate that flow. As a result, fresh Blood with healing nutrients is unable to reach the injured tissue.

I often see patients in agony from an intense stabbing form of back pain. Not able to find relief after making the rounds of various health professionals, they decide to try acupuncture. The sharp-knife symptoms usually mean Congealed Blood. Confirmed by physical examination, treatment will decongest the point of anguish and almost always provide immediate relief.

Lower back pain, though commonly due to sprain, also occurs from harmful climatic body invasions or Organ energy deficiency. Chinese Medicine recognizes how pathogenic elements intrude through the skin pores and settle in the lumbar and sacral regions of the back. The pathogenic culprit is mostly Damp Cold. By comparison, the Organ energy deficiency involved is Kidney Qi. Treatment addresses the cause. If Damp Cold proves to be the source, one must eliminate Damp Cold. On the other hand, Kidney deficiency needs strengthening.

Kidney energy requires special attention. It contains Inherited Energy or Essence, the life-supporting force we receive at birth from our parents. As we age, our Essence declines. It cannot be replaced, but it can be nourished and enhanced. Symptoms of the decrease show up as low back pain, knee pain, and arthritic conditions. Therapy involves relief for the painful area and general improvement of the Essence.

I really cannot stress enough the value of seeking answers in all available health services. One method of diagnosis and treatment may not hold the solution, but another will. Another could be less invasive and less expensive.

In cases of narrowing (spinal stenosis) or stiffening (ankylosing spondylitis), both the withering Organ energy and harmful invasions deserve evaluation. Bone degeneration reflects the lack of needed Blood and Qi for bone maintenance. As indicated, the acupuncturist is able to select modalities from a number of possibilities. Of course needling procedures, but additional help comes from electrical stimulation through the needles, suction cupping, herbal heat, and Chinese massage.

Baldness

Hair growth depends on Kidney Qi. Inherited tendencies usually account for male baldness. Kidney and Liver deficiencies also contribute to the problem, which is found less frequently in women. Needle combinations stimulate hair growth by energizing the Kidney and bringing Blood to the scalp. To help restore growth, you may try tapping your head with an apparatus called the seven star needle, a little flexible hammer that projects seven needles.

I suggest the herb Ho Shou Wu. Not only categorized as longevity medication, but it has indications to revive and darken hair. Many historic events and legends describe herbal discoveries. In this case, it seems that a man named Ho suffered illness since childhood, and as an adult always looked weak and deteriorated. By chance he came upon a plant that displayed a large number of flower blossoms. From its roots Ho prepared an edible herb, which he consumed over a year's time. Then people noticed his healthy appearance, but most notably his white hair had turned black. To honor Ho, the remedy was named Ho's Black Hair, or in Chinese Ho Shou Wu. The Latin name for the flowering plant is Polygonum multiflorum.

In general, I have observed better results in women with these methods. However, for years the herb has been part of my daily routine, and I always keep a full head of hair.

Bell's Palsy

Bell's palsy presents as paralysis of half the face including the eye. Pain may be involved. Western medicine remains puzzled regarding the cause, but thinks in terms of facial nerve compression. Therapy ordinarily uses steroids for pain and perhaps physical therapy for rehabilitation.

Acupuncture understands the exact source of the problem, an External Wind Invasion into Channels of the face. The mouth and eye deviate, the eye cannot close completely and the mouth has limitations for expression. When I studied in China, I observed and treated patients afflicted with a disorder called East Wind Invasion. It initially takes root in spring, but signs and symptoms develop in summer. Construction workers on buildings were the most prone, with outcomes similar to Bell's palsy.

Acupuncture on the face, head, upper and lower extremities, extracts Wind and improves circulation. Shown to be quite effective, certain needle combinations balance Wind disturbance with opposite, undisturbed facial parts. I feel that all cases of Bell's palsy ought to have referrals to acupuncturists.

Breast Cancer

Carcinoma of the breast continues to strike women at a growing rate. It causes more female fatalities then most other forms of malignancy. Examination and a mammogram can indicate a possible presence. Western medicine requires a biopsy for diagnosis.

Surgery, chemotherapy, and radiation therapy are frequent forms of treatment.

The lesion develops through stages. A movable soft lump in the breast with distinct covering defines a fibrous and cystic problem according to Western medicine. Chinese medicine interprets it as localized Phlegm. When harder but still movable, a layer of cells called the capsule has developed. This hardness indicates Phlegm with Blood Stagnation. A state where the lesion becomes more stationary suggests a malignant tumor to Western medicine, but Phlegm with Qi and Blood Stagnation to Chinese medicine.

China's medical literature described breast cancer hundreds of years ago. The cause was recognized as chronic negative emotions, particularly depression, anxiety, and pensive ways of thinking. Liver energy, which normally spreads evenly, turns increasingly inactive. No acupuncture points for needling exist on the breast, however, a major acupuncture Meridian runs through as the Stomach Channel. The Stomach, with its partner the Spleen, has much to do with worry, overburdening the mind while dwelling on persistent problems.

Today's active professional woman, who has enormous responsibilities, may overtax herself to the extent that her Stomach Channel becomes blocked. Acupuncture strengthens the emotions and prevents disease. It also effectively treats tumors, in the initial stages. Needling is applied to specific areas around the breast and at a distance to regulate the Stomach Channel. Herbal formulas for cancer also have proven helpful. A recommendation by the late Dr. James So of Boston, says clear the lesions first, before a biopsy.

At all stages, whether benign or malignant, acupuncture treats lesions in similar ways. Channels connected to the breast area require clearing, and normal circulation must be restored. The acupuncturist evaluates and treats Hot or Cold conditions. However, if the breast drains odorous fluid, the condition may not be treatable.

(See Cancer)

Breech Presentation of Fetus

At times, a prenatal situation occurs where the buttocks of the fetus, rather than the head, are positioned at the bottom of the uterus near the vaginal passage. Called breech presentation in obstetric speak, there is a risk dangerous for both mother and child, with a difficult delivery.

Applications of moxa heat to acupuncture points located on both feet correct the problem. This miraculously puts the baby in a normal position. When I perform this procedure with a few follow-up sessions, I observe the slight head protrusion, under the skin, move to its desired place. The other alternative is a Cesarean section (delivery through a surgical incision in the abdomen) or forced repositioning.

Bronchitis

Bronchitis produces coughs, fever, chills, sore throat, and uneasiness. Viral and bacterial infections are usually the cause, but weak immunity, smoking or air contaminants also contribute. Treatment largely employs antibiotics. Chronic bronchitis or chronic obstructive pulmonary disease (COPD), result from obstruction of airways, frequently with asthma or emphysema.

A number of acupuncture Lung patterns list symptoms of both acute and chronic bronchitis: Cold Violates Lung, Wind Heat Invades Lung, Lung Retains Damp Phlegm, Deficient Lung Qi, and Deficient Lung Yin. Treatment by acupuncture and herbs will remove the pathogenic elements or as needed, will strengthen the Lung and connected Organs.

(See Asthma)

Buerger's Disease

This peripheral vascular disease acts with inflammation on the smaller and medium size arteries and veins of the legs and arms. The source is attributed to cigarette smoking. Western medicine centers on specific anatomy, Chinese medicine considers Blood and Qi flow, Organ relationships, and Meridians. As an inflammatory process, a factor of Heat holds importance.

Burns

Acupuncture relieves the pain and aims to regenerate damaged tissues. An old remedy uses ginger juice and white wine directly on the burn, for which presently, you may substitute aloe gel. Ice application also helps.

Bursitis

Bursitis is inflammation of the bursa, which serve as lubricating sacs, particularly in regions of friction. These include places where tendons and muscles cross over bone protrusions and in joints. Terms such as tennis elbow, shoulder pain, Achilles tendon bursitis, bunion of the foot, and housemaid's knee depict common locations.

Western medicine in general remains uncertain as to the cause, but gives much attention to the exact structures afflicted and tissue changes. Injury, infection, and the inflammatory rheumatoid type of arthritis are some common causes. Doctors frequently prescribe steroid and nonsteroidal anti-inflammatory medications.

Chinese medicine looks at the different examples of bursitis as painful obstructions. In other words, Qi and Blood circulation has been blocked and pain emerges. Invasions of Wind, Cold, Damp, or Heat do their damage. Impairment by overuse weakens the body part, which becomes more susceptible to intruding harm. Kidney Qi rules bone and Liver Qi governs muscles, tendons, and ligaments. So flaws in these Organ energies also increase susceptibility.

Acupuncture eliminates the invading culprits, normalizes circulation, lubricates the joint, and strengthens Organ energy as needed. Of course, energy, pathologic forces and anatomy are integrated.

(See Foot Problems, Shoulder Pain and Tennis Elbow)

Cancer

A growing practice in China makes use of Western cancer diagnostic methods (i.e., blood tests, X-ray studies), but treats with acupuncture and herbs. Recently, a woman who is both a playwright and an actress came to my office with a complaint of liver cancer, diagnosed by medical laboratory findings. After a short series of visits in which I adjusted the Liver Qi and improved her emotions, she returned to her other doctor for reevaluation. To his surprise, all lab results showed no evidence of liver cancer. I have corrected cervical and various other cancers in much the same way.

When acupuncture or herbs cannot cure the malignancy, therapy tries to contain the disease, build up immunity and allow a lengthened period for survival with good quality of life. At times, acupuncture and herbs work with Western medicine's radiation, chemotherapy, and surgery. It may seem contradictory, since one principle of care attempts to balance energy and let the body heal itself. The other directly wants to kill the tumor. In spite of differences, coexistence with referrals on a mutually respectful basis will benefit the patient.

Two different approaches explain two concepts of cause. Western medicine considers geographic influences, inherited tendencies, viruses, environmental toxins, and deficiencies in the immune system. Chinese medicine leans more toward its traditional disease sources such as prolonged negative emotions, pathogenic invasions, Stagnation with toxic Heat, and ingestion of polluted food substances. Depending on the Organ or tissue involved, origins will vary as they relate to the form of cancer.

Treatment by acupuncture and herbs corresponds to the pathology. Positive emotions replace the negative, disease-producing invasions and toxins are released, and Stagnation becomes Activation of healthy energy.

Carpal Tunnel Syndrome

The carpal bones of the wrist form a tunnel, through which a nerve passes. Pressure on this nerve produces discomfort, distorted touch sensations, and weakness. Western medicine places the syndrome in the category of neuropathy (nerve disease).

Occupations that demand repeated overwork of the wrist, as well as some systemic diseases, bring it on. Splints and physical therapy may offer relief. The last resort is surgery.

I have found that acupuncture modalities offer improvement of the condition and often correction. There are acupuncturists who developed a specialization for the disorder. One modality employs a modified laser with success. My regimen combines acupuncture needling, moxa heat, and Chinese massage technique. Due to tightness and pain, I interpret it as a Cold Syndrome with Deficient or Blocked Qi.

I became afflicted with carpal tunnel symptoms, brought on by my acupuncture procedure work. Self-treatment eased the distress; however, significant help came to me through massage therapy. I bless my massage therapist.

Cigarette Addiction

Even though the health hazards of cigarette smoking have been greatly publicized, usage persists. Acupuncture proves to be quite effective to curb the addiction in most cases. In my practice, two to three sessions usually break the habit.

My associate from Beijing, Dr. Wan, had a special interest in addictions and taught me his methods. He addressed four phases in the rehabilitation process, all done by acupuncture. The first concerned relaxation, which needling easily accomplishes. Second, was mind control, meaning behavioral modification. This relates to the Chinese concept of the emotional Heart, through which we think. Third, he cleaned the Lungs with an application to energize Lung Qi. As a result, patients crave fresh air rather than smoke. Fourth, the addiction itself was treated using the ear. The Chinese see the ear as an extension of the Brain, thus messages go directly to the Brain from ear acupuncture. A tiny needle in a small patch of tape, attached to a specific ear point, continues the stimulation. These press pins are waterproof and are worn for a time.

Results have been very satisfying.

(See Addiction)

Cirrhosis

Commonly referred to as cirrhosis of the liver, the disease denotes pathologic changes of liver cells and tissues and the formation of nodules. Alcohol in excess, toxins, lack of nutritional protein, infection, and injury are causes. Jaundiced complexion and digestive upset typify signs and symptoms. Treatment includes dietary management and the elimination of alcohol intake.

Chinese medicine is in general agreement for the sources of this disease, but probes energy conditions rather than structure. The Organ energy most affected ties to the Spleen, and the adverse conditions are Damp and Heat for a Syndrome of Damp Heat Accumulates in Spleen. Digestion relies on Spleen Qi for the complete food absorption process. An overabundance of Heat obstructs bile to induce Jaundice.

In the rotation cycle of Organs, Liver should regulate Spleen. However, excesses in Spleen can back up and greatly disturb Liver. The source of the disorder still dwells in Spleen. To correct the problem, acupuncture gets rid of the Damp and Heat, and strengthens the Spleen.

Another illness relates to swelling or edema due to liver cirrhosis. Heart and intestinal disorders may accompany the Syndrome named Deficient Kidney Yang. Since Yang identifies Heat, this is a Cold condition with excess fluid. Systemic abnormal states will act upon many areas in the body. This case involves Cold, therefore, chills, cold back, cold knees, and a pale face complexion becomes apparent. Instead of Damp Heat, it is Damp Cold.

Cirrhosis connects to Western medicine through structural evaluation of the liver. Depending on signs and symptoms, Chinese medicine cares for the Spleen or the Kidney. For improvement, it rejects Spleen Damp Heat and enhances Kidney Yang.

Although one affects the other, we are dealing with comparisons of visual organ pathology and the unseen dimension of Organ Qi.

Colic

This usually describes abdominal pain during infancy with incessant crying. Common in children are food accumulation disorders that yield Heat. The digestive build-up causes discomfort and the Heat leads to irritability and sleeplessness.

Simple needling frees the abundance and lowers Heat. I have effectively treated a colicky baby as young as ten days old.

Colitis

As an inflammation of the intestine with diarrhea, Western medicine usually links it to pathogenic organisms or emotional stress. Symptoms include abdominal pain, blood and pus in the stool, and fever. Dysentery, a more serious inflammation with overlapping symptoms, occurs with infections of bacteria, viruses, amoebae, and toxins.

In Chinese medicine, the colitis Syndrome is Damp Heat in the Large Intestine. Elimination of the two troublemakers, Damp and Heat, should solve the problem. Acute dysentery reflects a Hot condition, if chronic it means Cold.

Coma

States of unconsciousness differ from a momentary stupor where immediate arousal is possible, to a serious coma, when the patient shows no response at all. We find reasons for the lack of alertness in brain dysfunction. These include tumors, infection, bleeding, injury, toxins, lack of oxygen, diabetes, and epilepsy or abnormal psychiatric behavior.

According to Chinese medicine, the Heart contains the Spirit and houses the Mind. It governs speech and maintains consciousness and memory. In other words, we think with our Heart and we speak with our emotions. The closely attached Organ, the Pericardium, surrounds and protects the Heart. The protector also absorbs excesses. They work together.

By comparison, the Brain has more to do with the spinal cord, Kidney and Essence. A strong Brain supports mental focus and vision. The Heart operates with emotional Spirit; the Brain with practical Essence. A substandard state of awareness points to a Heart disorder.

The intrusion of two pathogenic elements on Heart activity, namely Heat and Phlegm, overcome a person, causing a lapse into a stupor or coma. Various degrees of mental illness result from Phlegm misting Heart openings. A severe case of excess leads to unconsciousness. For recovery, the Spleen has a major function, as it can resolve Phlegm. The Heart itself also requires a boost.

Heat that falls into the Pericardium can bring about mental illness, delirium, and coma. Emergency care calms the Heart and releases the Heat. Needle bloodletting procedures prove life saving. One day a computer repairman inhaled chemical fumes while working in my office. He had a reaction, turned hot and started to drift into a comatose state. I immediately bled points on his hands, which drained the Heat and restored full consciousness.

Common Cold

Western medicine has identified several viruses associated with the common cold. Bacteria can complicate the condition. Typical of the ailment are symptoms of coughing, sneezing, runny nose, and sore throat. Inflammation appears in the nose, the adjacent sinuses, throat, and possibly lungs. Decongestants and pain medications are recommended with rest. Steam inhalation may assist respiration.

In contrast, acupuncture examines consequences of pathogenic invasions of Wind either with Cold or Heat. Granted, germs may find the unhealthy internal environment as habitable, but the problem exists in the environment, in the Lung. When Cold invades the Lung, a little fever with chills and body ache occur followed by a runny or stuffy nose and coughing. Care with acupuncture and herbs abolish Cold and Wind and the common cold. Of course, The Lung must increase in strength.

Wind Heat invasion creates a more severe fever, heavy yellow phlegm, perspiration, and perhaps a bleeding nose. Treatment will reduce the excess Heat and get rid of the Wind.

(See Influenza)

Conjunctivitis

Inflammation of the conjunctivae, the mucous membranes that line the eyelids, is named conjunctivitis. Viruses, bacteria, allergies or air irritants may induce the disorder. Antibiotic drops or ointment with or without steroids can alleviate the condition.

Acupuncture considers two sources, one external and the other internal. Invading Wind Heat penetrates and brings on inflammation. The internal disease process originates in the Liver from which strong Heat or Fire rises. This also prompts high blood pressure and migraine headaches. But Liver energy's inclination always travels up to and opens in the eye.

Application of specific needling drives out Wind Heat and improves ocular circulation. A different approach with acupuncture anchors the Rising Liver Fire and encourages the Yin to cool things down. Both treatments usually correct the disease at hand.

(See Eye Ailments)

Coronary Artery Disease

Coronary artery vessels supply blood to the heart itself. The heart is a muscle known as the myocardium. Coronary artery disease prevents sufficient blood from reaching the myocardium due to narrowing of the vessels. Related conditions include angina pectoris, resulting from insufficient oxygen, and a myocardial infarction, which is a sudden lack of blood to one area of the heart. Medication and surgery are common treatments.

In Chinese medicine, these disorders fit into a category of Heart pain. The course of disease follows deficient strength of the Heart or specifically Deficient Yang of the Heart.

Another Syndrome involves Blood Stagnation, which could have a complication of Damp Phlegm. As indicated, invigoration of Yang, or of Blood Stagnation, and removal of Phlegm will heal the sick Heart.

Cushing's Disease and Addison's Disease

Excess secretion of the adrenal metabolic hormone called cortisol describes Cushing's disease. A prominent sign appears as a rounded moon face. The opposite condition is Addison's disease where a deficiency of the hormone disrupts metabolism and there is increased skin pigmentation, with weakness and fatigue.

Since the adrenal glands sit on the kidneys, Kidney energy bestows on them a powerful influence. Regulating Kidney may normalize the overflow and invigorating Kidney may restore hormonal secretion. This shows an example of acupuncture's ability in energy to work with body chemistry.

Cystic Fibrosis

I will never forget the day a mother came into the office carrying her ten-year-old son in her arms. She said to me that she wanted her son back. Diagnosed with cystic fibrosis at age six, he was just discharged from an extended stay in a local hospital for the treatment of a respiratory infection, consisting of intravenous antibiotics. The boy became very weak. However, until now he was very physically active and mentally alert. I assured the mother I would do everything possible to help her son.

We share so many diseases, which China has treated by acupuncture since ancient times. Unfortunately, not included is cystic fibrosis. As an inherited gastrointestinal and respiratory condition, mucous plugs develop in the lungs and pancreas, and excess sodium and chloride are secreted in perspiration. I made comparisons with bronchial asthma, which is certainly not as severe. Yet, asthma does hold a similar origin in Deficient or Disturbed Lung, Spleen or Kidney Qi. Phlegm, wheezing, coughing, and shortness of breath occur as comparable symptoms. Children with cystic fibrosis often display strong fevers, not exhibited in asthma.

Using asthma as my treatment model, with variations as indicated in acupuncture and herbal formulas, much improvement came to pass. Soon a CAT scan of the lungs revealed no mucous plugs, while symptoms disappeared. A year later, there was normal body growth and plenty of participation in sports. The mother said he had a burst of energy.

I presented my research on this disease in the American Journal of Acupuncture, discussing possible reasons why China's population lacks cystic fibrosis. For centuries, the Chinese have pursued enhancement of their Inherited Qi or Essence, which could heighten healthier reproductive qualities. From early childhood, infants receive treatment to normalize digestion and suppress Phlegm accumulations. The traditional Chinese diet remains dairy-free after breast-feeding. Another factor may relate to Chinese medicine's leanings to natural therapy.

Trying to find answers to life-threatening diseases spends millions of dollars and consumes endless hours of research. I sincerely believe that solutions may conceivably present themselves through research in Chinese medicine. We must put forth the effort.

Deafness

Western medicine searches for sources of deafness either from a lesion in one of two hearing (auditory) canals or on the eighth cranial nerve. The eighth cranial nerve is one of twelve nerve pairs that originate in the brain and connects to sensory functions in the head such as vision, smell, taste and hearing. A few of the nerves also control structural movement and facial expression. A tuning fork and other sound conduction tests offer data for evaluation. Injury and infection are additional possibilities. Often ringing in the ear called tinnitus precedes hearing loss.

Drainage, excision and incision procedures, antibiotics, and drops in the ear routinely treat the ailments. There may be defects from birth or loss with aging, requiring a hearing aid.

Organ energies travel to and open on parts of the head. Liver opens at the eyes, Lung in the nose, Spleen through the mouth, Heart in the tongue, and Kidney at the ears. Kidney, the holder of Essence, may have deficiencies that prevent enough Qi and Blood from supporting hearing abilities. Spleen Deficiency can cause similar trouble. Also, excess Heat in the Liver rises through Gallbladder Channels that surround the ear. Overweight patients could be prone to Heat and Phlegm Stagnation, interfering with hearing. Many reasons exist for this sensory loss.

The Qi disturbances probably involve lesions and infection, but an understanding in the energy dimension just may correct the hearing disorder. Acupuncture clears the congestion and regulates related Organ imbalances.

Dermatitis

Dermatitis means inflammation of the skin, often with redness, itching, and various kinds of lesions. The terms eczema and dermatitis are usually interchangeable. Adjectives can describe specifics in dermatitis, for example, allergic dermatitis comes from an allergy, atopic dermatitis has an unknown cause but contact dermatitis touches upon a specific irritant like a perfume or soap.

When I studied dermatology during my hospital residency, the dermatologist routinely prescribed an antihistamine by mouth and cortisone cream for the skin. A complication of an infection would demand antibiotics. Together, the medications usually helped his patients.

Chinese medicine interprets skin invasions of Heat, Wind, and Damp. Heat gives rise to inflammation, Wind produces itching and Damp-Heat creates a basis for infection. Certain acupuncture points direct an indicated healing reaction. Intestinal toxins may

101

surface to form a skin problem. Therefore, a major skin-center point strengthens the Large Intestine. Two Spleen connected points are frequently used in dermatology, one regulates Blood and the other releases excess Damp. A couple of insertions will eliminate Wind. The immune system, or in Chinese medicine language, the Protective Qi at the skin surface, ought to be fortified.

I treat many skin disorders often through a combination of acupuncture and herbs. They usually lead to gratifying results.

(See Acne, Shingles)

Diabetes

Inadequate insulin production by the pancreas organ produces diabetes. Typical symptoms include increased thirst, hunger, and urination. Laboratory testing finds elevated blood sugar. Eventually other complications such as abnormal circulatory and nerve function (neuropathy) may arise. Treatment consists of diet and insulin replacement. Two classes of diabetes indicate the need for insulin. Type I has a vital dependence on insulin for survival. Type II does not require the insulin substitute to maintain life, but may use it to control symptoms.

Chinese medicine takes a different approach and attempts to cure the disease. It sees the body's internal environment as generating too much Heat by three pathways: (1) by the ingestion of fatty, rich meals and large amounts of alcohol, the Spleen and Stomach suffer and so does digestive assimilation. Food breakdown Stagnates, which induces excessive Heat; (2) prolonged negative emotions also yield Stagnation. Stagnant Qi then turns to Fire; and (3) exhausting physical activities or a lingering Warm element can harm Kidney Yin, causing Heat and diabetes. These three Heat-producing sequences also occur in juvenile diabetes.

The Heat evaporates fluid to include insulin causing symptoms of thirst to follow Lung affliction; of hunger, Stomach; of urination, Kidney. Treatment removes Heat, normalizes Organs and restores Kidney Yin.

Down's Syndrome

This represents a genetic disorder of retardation of physical and mental development in children. It's due to an extra chromosome that has been discovered in the cell nucleus. Associated signs appear as a sloping forehead, slanted eyes, flat nose, a single crease in the palm and a small body size. Care for the little one, consists of health maintenance.

Progress with acupuncture therapy in China offers us an alternative. If begun before three years of age, correction starts to take place. After three, doctors find limitations. Deficiencies in Inherited and uterine Qi, and Blood, are at the root of the defect. After delivery, deficiency in nutrition due to Spleen and Kidney weakness remains a factor.

Applications of acupuncture strive to build up the Brain and spinal cord, and Qi and Blood circulation. A number of the points have their locations on the head.

Drug Addiction

Addiction to drugs progresses with serious consequences. Family members make appointments at my office for young addicted relatives.

Much of the treatment focuses on the ear, which exerts a

powerful force on the Brain and body in general. The ear serves as an extension of the Brain and, in miniature, represents the entire body.

Stimulated points relax the patient, curtail the addiction and manage the autonomic nervous system. Deep Organ energies are enhanced. I try to increase emotional strength as much as possible with head and body needling.

Follow-up sessions reach higher levels of correction. A series of visits give the best result.

(See Addiction)

Chapter 8
Ear Infection to Knee Pain

Ear Infection

Blockages and various forms of ear congestion occur in both children and adults. Antibiotics cure infection. Tumors and injuries are also causes. Some of these problems do not respond to treatment resulting in chronic conditions.

In Chinese medicine, Kidney energy opens to the ear. Deficient Yin of Kidney gives rise to overflowing empty Yang Heat, the source of chronic disorders. A Yin-Yang balance in turn shows promise for correction.

Channel energies from certain Organs surround the ear and can cause or cure problems. They are made up of the Gallbladder, Small Intestine, and Triple Warmer. The Triple Burner in itself represents three functional regions of Organs in the torso. Acupuncture stimulates the Channel locally around the ear and at a distance, for example on the hand. Chronic drainage from infection receives help too, by herbal remedies.

(See Deafness, Meniere's Disease, Tinnitus)

Eczema
(See Dermatitis)

Edema

Abnormal amounts of fluids can accumulate in the body as a whole or in a specific area. This swelling known as edema may occur for multiple reasons. Weakened small blood vessels with increased pressure, obstruction, heart, kidney or liver failure, and body chemical or hormonal imbalances are a few. Depending on the cause, Western therapy may restrict fluid intake and salt, and if indicated, prescribe a diuretic.

Chinese medicine emphasizes responsibility of Organ Qi. The Spleen controls the production of Body Fluids from metabolized food and drink; the Lung regulates water passages; the Kidney is the driving force by supplying the Spleen with Yang Heat to transform fluids, otherwise they stagnate, accumulate and swell. Even in swollen (edematous) pulmonary heart disease, the Heart and Kidney Yang demand attention.

Elbow Pain

Overuse related to work or sports, disturbs and blocks local circulation. Acupuncture, most often with moxa heat, restores a healthy Blood and Qi flow.

(See Bursitis, Tennis Elbow)

Emergencies

Many more lives could be saved by the incorporation of acupuncture. Loss of consciousness, no matter what the source, calls for reviving needle techniques. We should do everything possible to save a life; for example, a certain acupuncture point treats drowning.

(See Coma, Heart Problems, and Stroke)

Emotions

Emotions are invisible forces of energy of which Chinese medicine takes a deep and active interest. Like other energies, they cannot be seen but can be felt. What can be seen however, are their effects on the human body, the complexion, the expression, and the sparkle in the eye. When negative and constant, physical signs and symptoms of disorders directly mirror the bad tempered feelings. Prolonged negative emotions cause diseases. For example, depression lowers immunity allowing illness to take root.

From centuries of diagnostic experience, acupuncture has learned to match sensitivity to an Organ. On my initial doctor-patient consultation, I often ask what is the emotion experienced during stress. People subjectively know what they feel. This clues me in regarding the disease source and associated physical problems.

There are seven classic emotional states: anger, joy, worry, sadness, grief, fear, and fright. Based on similarities, sadness is combined with grief, and fear with fright or shock. Liver attaches to anger, also depression and frustration; Heart to joy, Spleen to worry, Lung to sadness, and Kidney to fear and anxiety. A percentage of my patients present no physical ailments, only psychological issues.

For each negative emotion there exists a positive one. The

goal in acupuncture therapy is to reconstruct a positive direction. Anger changes to a healthy aggressiveness. Every emotion involves the Heart, but primarily the range covers joyful, overjoyed, and hysterical moods. Heat accumulates in the Heart; the more the Fire increases the more serious the condition. Cooling and calming the Heart will benefit emotions. In addition, worry changes to insightful intelligence, sadness to empathy, and fear to courage.

Emphysema

As a chronic lung disease, emphysema develops from a loss of elasticity and distention of lung tissue. Causes connect to cigarette smoking and environmental air pollution. Avoidance is recommended with symptomatic treatment.

Chinese medicine thinks in terms of Deficient Lung Qi. Treatment attempts to energize the Lung and work through the Spleen to eliminate Phlegm.

Endometriosis

The inner lining of the uterus is called the endometrium. For new life, a fertilized ovum (reproductive cell) implants itself in this mucous membrane lining. When the endometrium fixes itself outside the uterus, it is called endometriosis. Symptoms frequently result as menstrual or pelvic pain, and infertility. Medication to suppress the growth and surgical removal offer a correction as the usual forms of treatment.

The Chinese designation of uterine mass references Stagnation, either of Blood, with Heat or due to Cold. Acupuncture treats and reverses the disease process. Relief of symptoms should follow.

Eye Ailments

Through certain acupuncture points, many eye disorders do well. Needle stimulation lubricates, alleviating dryness, reduces excess tears, drains congestion and restores Blood and Qi circulation. Liver energy opens to the eyes and may be the basic source of problems, particularly when related to stress or eyestrain. Pressure at work or school while overusing your eyes, at times reduces the Yin of the Liver, which lets the Yang rise to the head. Sparks before the eyes develop, often accompanied by a migraine headache.

Invasions with Wind also stir up trouble. Wind Heat blown into the head obstructs circulation and fails to bring nourishment into and around the eye. Squinting (strabismus) could also be an outcome, caused by an internal circulatory weakness. Crossed eyes in childhood present similar signs, possibly due to persistent Heat.

A combination of anger-induced ascending Liver Fire with a Wind invasion could produce sudden visual failure. In addition, Gall Bladder Channels that surround the eyes take in the Heat. This emergency and the other ailments listed above usually react favorably to acupuncture.

Cataracts, if treated early enough, may attain a cure. However, once the lens has thickened and becomes opaque, acupuncture has limitations and I recommend surgery. I have an ophthalmologist friend who performs cataract correcting surgery with wonderful results.

There are three Deficiency ailments: optic atrophy (degeneration of the optic nerve), macular degeneration (degeneration of the retina's center, the nerve network in back of the eye that constitutes the retina), and retinitis pigmentosa (progressive loss of peripheral vision followed by tunnel vision). These are all medical words for disorders that Chinese medicine regard as energy deficiencies and related Organ imbalances. Deficiencies in fact take place in the aging nervous system.

Help from acupuncture restores Qi and regulates Liver, Kidney, Spleen or Heart connections. Fresh Blood and Qi must nourish the eyes.

Glaucoma is associated with increased pressure in the eye and varying degrees of vision impairment. Wide ranges of diagnostic categories describe abnormal structure and symptoms. Depending on the exact evaluation, treatments include eye drops, oral medication, or laser surgery.

Of course, Chinese medicine evaluates the energy dimension, with concern for emotional factors. These relate to disharmonies of the Heart. Abnormal Liver function also plays a major role, moving pathogenic elements upward. Systemic weaknesses focus on the Kidney. In general, I have found satisfactory results by draining glaucoma congestion downward to the foot.

A consideration in eye care relates to other systemic diseases such as diabetes. Injury remains another factor, but the greatest attention focuses on the Liver. Liver dysfunction is very much reflected in eye dysfunction.

(See Conjunctivitis)

Fertility

Inability to conceive presents a major problem for many couples who desire children. Insufficient male sperm, dysfunction of the ovaries or the fallopian tubes are possible causes. Additional explanations focus on abnormal structures of the uterus, cysts, tumors, infections, and hormonal disorders. When examination reveals no abnormalities, the option of in vitro fertilization—from husband or a donor—offers a solution.

China is the most populous country in the world. They must be doing something right. Indeed, for millennia their medicine has studied sex and reproduction. I am not always successful, but have achieved conception with acupuncture after other methods have failed. Traditional herbal medication supplements the acupuncture.

Chinese medicine theory of male infertility focuses on deficient Kidney Qi in decreased sexual energy and Damp Heat in the Liver interfering with male function.

Female reproductive weaknesses could stem from Stagnant Blood, Deficiencies or Excesses in an energy Channel that surrounds the waistline, also Cold in the Uterus or too much Cold or Heat in the Pelvic area. Following an evaluation, acupuncture pursues normalcy by correcting the defects such as irregular menstrual periods.

States of stress and prolonged negativity influence reproduction. In my experience, conception at times follows acupuncture's application to increase emotional strength. Consultation that goes beyond questions of symptoms, but includes deep, inner feelings becomes important. The physical and mental can receive treatment at the same time.

I have had good results working with fertility clinics. Applied before and after in vitro procedures, acupuncture maintains reproductive energy. Patients with tendencies to miscarry are treated until delivery. This is another example where Chinese and Western medicine, together, can benefit the patient.

Fever

A rise in body temperature as shown by thermometer readings

indicates fever. Infections will induce it, plus other ailments including dehydration, certain skin diseases, irregular heart and vascular functions, cerebral bleeding, rheumatoid arthritis, and drug reactions. Some febrile episodes have unknown causes. This is where acupuncture comes in to identify and treat all types of Fever.

A Yin-Yang imbalance in Organs—lowered cool Yin and increased hot Yang—elevates body Heat. Ordinarily, Deficient Yin takes place within the Lung, Heart, Kidney, and Liver. Excess Heat, often with Dampness, can penetrate the Lung, Heart, Pericardium, Liver, Gall Bladder, Large Intestine, and Urinary Bladder. Heat Invasions produce Fever as they move deeper into the body by stages. Lesser Heat appears from a Cold attack, where the body's warm defenses take action.

Fibromyalgia

A relatively new disease entity, fibromyalgia means pain in the muscles and connective tissues. Identified by points of tenderness, and thought to originate from injury, cold, damp, toxins, physical and mental stress, treatment recommendations lean toward natural therapies. Muscle stretching, massage and heat applications may help. Treatment may also consist of anesthetic and steroid injections.

Assessments by acupuncturists bear in mind symptoms of Circulatory Blockages, since the Chinese word for pain frequently translates as Blockage pain. My observations interpret Cold, Damp and Congealed Blood. Clearing Obstacles and restoring a smooth Blood Flow is a treatment goal.

A middle-aged woman recently came to my office, diagnosed with fibromyalgia. Her complaints consisted of sharp stabbing pain in the back and a painful stiff neck, both of long duration. After consultation and examination, I made an acupuncture diagnosis of Congealed Blood in the back and Cold Blockages of the neck. Obviously, Cold contracts and stiffens.

I then released the Congealed Blood and drained Obstructions from the neck using needles, cupping, and herbal heat. The patient felt immediate relief. After a total of four visits, she was cured of the disorder. Not everyone responds the same; some require many treatments and some very few.

Foot Problems

As a former doctor of podiatric medicine, I am very familiar with disorders of the feet. Many respond well to acupuncture needling. Structural deformity, of course, may need mechanical orthotic supports or surgical repair. It has been my experience that injuries, poor surgical outcomes, and vascular diseases do improve in numerous cases, with acupuncture.

A bunion refers to a bursitis at the joint behind the large toe. Common practices employ steroid injections, protective padding, or surgery. Passing through the bunion is an energy Channel. Acupuncture regulates this Meridian to relieve the bunion pain. Comparable treatment applies to hammer toes.

Heel pain frequently involves a heel spur, probably due to pulling of an attached fibrous band called the plantar fascia. Steroid injections, fitted orthotics or surgery are current methods of therapy. Chinese medicine does not emphasize the irregular structure, but instead focuses on bone pain from Circulatory Blockage. Kidney related points in the area are needled, because Kidney energy controls bone. In addition, deep acupuncture at tender spots, I find greatly eliminates discomfort.

Ulcers (open sores) on the foot often develop as a complication of diabetes. Energy attracts Blood. When needle simulation brings in Qi, Blood will follow with its nutrients to close and cure an ulcer. We are thus helping the body to heal itself. I have prevented amputations by this method.

Gallstones

Stones form in the gallbladder or related ducts in huge numbers of people. Many undergo surgical removal of the gallbladder. Another approach chemically dissolves stones by medication. Age, excess weight, heredity, and diet all contribute to the condition.

According to Chinese medical principles, the even Flow of Qi and Blood are attributed to Liver function. It works closely with the Gallbladder, which stores and secretes bile. It also aids digestion in the Spleen and Stomach when moving smoothly. Damp Heat and a prolonged negative emotion like anger will hinder the action of Liver Qi that affects bile as well. Then the constrained bile hardens into stones. Stagnant Stomach Qi, from irregular Liver function, adds to the formation of gallstones.

Acupuncture technique removes Damp Heat and Stagnancy. It also will reenergize Liver and Stomach. In China, ear therapy works effectively. The ear serves as a micro-acupuncture system that represents the entire body in miniature. Stimulation on points associated with Organs, for example, Liver, Gall Bladder, Stomach, Spleen, and others have shown success. Often, practitioners fasten a type of seed, rather than a needle, to the outer ear with a tape adhesive.

Gastritis (Stomach Inflammation)

Western medicine searches for abnormal changes in the stomach lining in connection to symptoms of pain, tenderness on pressure, nausea or vomiting. One condition is gastric or peptic ulcers, which can develop in the presence of certain bacteria. Excess stomach acid has much importance, especially when treated. Still, uncertainties exist as to causes.

Chinese medicine gives its full attention to subjective symptoms. Differentiation is made between Cold or Hot diseases or Stagnation. Cold in the Stomach, from too much cold food, exhibits severe pain, but also a systemic Cold condition with Cold hands and Cold feet. After an illness, Stomach and Spleen Yang may decrease to yield Cold ulcers.

Damp Heat in the Spleen could result in acute gastritis. Furthermore, we have Blazing Fire in the Stomach with extreme Dryness, and Congealed Blood in the Stomach that produces a stabbing pain and bloated abdomen. Liver Stagnation is another entity.

Acupuncture treatment for each of these ailments must concentrate on restoring balance. Warm a Cold disorder, remove Damp Heat, cool down extreme Heat, disperse Congealed Blood and activate Stagnation.

Goiter

Goiter is an enlarged thyroid gland in the neck. Therapy consists of administration of thyroid hormone. Acupuncture distinguishes a sequence of events. At first, depressed emotions lead to Liver Qi Stagnation, which eventually heats up and generates Phlegm and Blood stasis. Together they form a goiter. Treatment cools the Fire, gets rid of the Phlegm, moves the Stagnation and vitalizes the Qi. Goiter and hyperthyroidism are treated in the same way.

Heart Problems

Both Chinese and Western medicine standards understand the heart's role in blood circulation. Both cultures additionally perceive an emotional association. Expressed in our language, for example, if you love someone, you love with all your heart, not all your liver. Nonetheless, the Chinese have documented many more functions. The Heart holds the Spirit and Mind, therefore, we think, talk, and sleep by way of our Heart. Within this Organ, we provide care for alertness, memory, speech and a night's rest.

Deficiencies of Blood, Qi, Yin or Yang, and Blood Stagnation, serve as grounds for various Western diagnoses that include arrhythmia, cardiac insufficiency, and infarctions (degenerated areas). By regulating the disharmonies, better Heart function returns. Because of the linkage, care of the Heart includes the emotions and care of the emotions includes the Heart.

The Kidney, symbolized by Water, controls the Heart, symbolized by Fire. At times, a cardiac disorder can stem from the Kidney. In reverse, as a diseased heart weakens, kidney failure follows. This is regularly documented in our Western hospitals.

(See Angina Pectoris, Coronary Artery Disease)

Hemorrhoids

Varicose veins in the rectal area are known as external or internal hemorrhoids. They can bleed, protrude and cause pain. Management of the condition uses injections, ointments, banding (ligation), or surgical removal.

There is a Qi that holds Blood and Organs in their place. When unable to do the job, the energy drops down. The supporting force works as Spleen Qi. Although needling to strengthen the Spleen proves helpful, exact indicated points further reduce hemorrhoids. One exists on top of the head, which raises Qi in general, others on the arms, legs and low back. Also, applications of moxa heat benefit the patient.

During my hospital residency, I remember a staff physician who suffered from recurrent hemorrhoids. Multiple surgeries were not able to correct the annoying condition. Of course, only structure was considered, no one knew about Spleen Qi.

Hepatitis

Defined as inflammation of the liver, hepatitis is often associated with jaundice. It can be acute or chronic. Viruses, alcohol, and toxins have been recognized as some causes. There is no direct corrective treatment. Chinese medicine points to the internal Damp environment that harbors the virus or toxin.

The pathogenic factor is based on Damp Heat. Damp Heat of the Spleen brings on an acute infection. When of the Gall Bladder, a brighter colored jaundice appears. In both the Liver and Gall Bladder, it is a more serious, infectious hepatitis than that of just the Spleen. Acupuncture, with protective caution, resolves the Damp and eliminates the Heat. An important application builds up the afflicted Organ's vitality and immunity.

Hernia

Hernia refers to a protrusion of an organ through a containing wall. Treatment positions the projection back in place by surgical

117

sutures or by a restraining device known as a truss. Acupuncture activates an extra Meridian that penetrates through all solid or Yin Organs. Beneficial in the acute stage of hernia, it's employed also for a prolapsed uterus in women. Then selections from a number of points in and around the hernia region energize containment.

(See Prolapse of Uterus and Rectum)

High Blood Pressure and Hypertension

Hypertension arises from very high blood pressure with different symptoms. These could manifest as dizziness, headache, bloody nose, reddish face, and irritability. Causes are stress, hereditary, arteriosclerosis, hormonal, renal, and a great deal of unknowns.

Chinese medicine considers hypertension a symptom of impaired Organs. For example, heavy Phlegm in the upper body can initiate the distressful condition. Regulating Spleen Qi, in turn, expels the Phlegm. Deficiency of Heart Blood or Yin, and Deficient Kidney Yin, creates the problem as well. Liver disharmonies provide a source in Rising Liver Yang or Fire, and Liver Yin Deficiency. Each syndrome requires a diagnostic evaluation based on symptoms, emotions, and examination of the tongue and pulse. Once a pattern has been established, acupuncture reverses the disease process.

Hip Disorders

The hip may sustain fractures, dislocations, and degeneration. Surgical pinning or joint replacements are standard procedure. I have performed acupuncture before and after surgery, which speeds healing.

A method to regenerate bone in this region uses needle stimulation along a meridian on the side of the thigh, hip and low back. In the upper back, two points control the energy center of bone for anyplace on the body. A woman in her forties was scheduled for a hip replacement due to pain and degeneration seen on X-ray studies. Through clearing of the relevant Meridians, to restore healthy circulation and activate the center of bone energy, regeneration took place and the surgery was canceled.

(See Arthritis)

Hyperthyroidism

To Western medicine, hyperthyroidism is an excess thyroid secretion disease with metabolic demands and a goiter as a sign. In Chinese medicine, hyperthyroidism and goiter are comparable. Both recognize the presence of Heat, irregular emotions, insomnia, perspiration, heart palpitations, protruding eyes, hunger, and thirst. Iodine prevents a simple goiter. Radiation therapy and surgical removal are treatment options. Energy patterns that induce an enlarged thyroid are Deficient Heart Blood and the Heat yielding Deficient Heart Yin, and Stomach Fire.

Hypothyroidism, deficient thyroid secretion, does not appear in traditional Chinese medical literature. However, acupuncture today can regulate and treat this thyroid disorder.

(See Goiter)

Incontinence

Urinary incontinence is the failure to retain urine. The involuntary incident varies in degree and situations. Sometimes pressure on the abdomen, stress, or a sneeze and cough will bring it on. Factors range from bladder infection, blockages, weaknesses, and lesions to systemic disease such as multiple sclerosis. For treatment, there are medications and surgery.

Energy patterns give a different insight. A disease process called Spleen Qi Sinking produces the dysfunction. Strengthening and raising Spleen Qi by acupuncture will reduce the defect. Other causes exist in Deficient Kidney Essence (Inherited Qi) and Deficient Bladder Qi. Vitalizing the respective Organs should improve the condition.

(See Urinary Problems)

Indigestion

Digestion that falls short of a completely smooth process occurs with nausea, vomiting, heartburn, reflux discomfort, bloating, and gas. It is often a challenge to diagnose, especially when physical abnormalities are not found. Then, attention looks toward psychological issues as the basis for gastrointestinal upsets. Western and Chinese medicine share some agreement regarding emotions as seen in expressions such as "I can't stomach him" and "I hate his guts".

The emotional associations in acupuncture encompass anger and frustration. They cause Stagnation of Liver energy and decrease food absorption. Stomach and Spleen react in a negative way to worry.

Chinese advice warns against the ingestion of too much cold food. Cold in the Spleen and Large Intestine results in symptoms of indigestion. It must be noted that the Spleen has a major role in the assimilation of food.

Rebellious Stomach Qi emerges from Stagnation. Normally, Stomach Qi descends. If it rises, one experiences nausea, vomiting, hiccup, and related symptoms. Food Stagnation in children becomes detrimental, since the digestive system matures while digestion continues.

All these anomalies respond to acupuncture application. One combination of needles regulates the entire digestive system. There is a technique that draws down and drains Stomach excesses. Moxa heat effectively warms a Cold Stomach problem. At the same time, psychological weaknesses gain strength.

(See Gastritis, Reflux)

Infection

Bacteria, viruses, fungus and parasites cause infection. Classic symptoms list pain, heat, redness and swelling, in other words, the same description for inflammation but without the bugs. Infection may be localized or widespread. Acupuncture focuses on the unfavorable setting that welcomes toxins and Damp Heat.

Western medicine aims to kill the pathogenic microorganisms, or weaken them and let the immune system finish the job. Acupuncture restores a healthy internal environment where infection cannot develop and flourish.

(See Abscess)

Influenza

Influenza, customarily known as the flu, in acupuncture enters the same category as the common cold. Our medicine emphasizes a pathogenic virus for flu, and virus or bacteria for a cold. The Chinese concept of the unhealthy internal environment applies to both ailments. Wind Cold or Wind Heat in the Lung could become complicated with Phlegm. Treatment disperses the Wind, Cold or Heat and expels the Phlegm.

(See Common Cold)

Insomnia

Inadequate sleep due to periods of interruption, pain, systemic disease, anxiety or depression, meet Western medicine's criteria for evaluations of sleeplessness. Aging has also shown to change snooze patterns. Hypnotic pills and traditional suggestions from fresh air exercise to drinking a glass of warm milk may ease someone off to a night's rest.

Chinese medicine makes different observations. During the day, Qi flows through the outer Yang Meridians, and at night, the inner Yin Meridians. In addition, sleepy time Yang penetrates deeply and Yin surfaces. That is why we like to have a covering after dark, to warm us in the cool Yin. A Yin-Yang imbalance with excess emerging Yang Heat while trying to sleep keeps us awake. The Heat can even dilate skin pores and cause night sweats. Decreasing the night Yang and increasing the night Yin will remedy the insomnia.

The Heart controls sleep. If unable to fall asleep, it often means the Heart lacks sufficient Blood. Therefore, replenished Blood to the Heart ought to correct the problem. During the office visit, I always calm the emotions and include specific resting points. Popular in China, two points behind the head at the base of the scalp, translate as "restful sleep I" and "restful sleep II".

Rising Liver Fire (Hot Yang) results in insomnia as well. Treatment certainly would stabilize Liver Qi, cool the Yang and correct the aggravating emotion.

Irritable Bowel Syndrome (IBS)

Constipation, diarrhea, diverse types of abdominal pain, and fluctuation of bowel movements, characterize irritable bowel syndrome or IBS. One kind reacts with pain from eating; another type stays pain free but strikes with diarrhea urgency. Western medicine cannot find any definite structural abnormality, but feels that an emotional stress factor ties in. People may experience symptoms of nausea, gas, abdominal bloating and discomfort, headache, and thought disturbances. Patient care includes psychological support and dietary recommendations.

Acupuncturists try to fit a Western syndrome to an established Chinese syndrome. This pattern comes close to Deficient Qi of the Large Intestine. Urgent diarrhea suggests Damp Heat. Intense pain points to Stagnation. The emotions are treated as needed.

I have actually achieved good results by relieving the particular symptoms and adjusting the Large Intestine Qi. Combinations of needle technique bring about a more normal regularity.

(See Indigestion)

Jaundice

Chinese and Western medicine agree that jaundice appears as a sign for an underlying disease. They both acknowledge how the yellowish skin color will diminish upon correction of the internal sickness. Usually it signals a faulty liver with bile obstruction.

Acupuncture views jaundice as an accumulation of Dampness in certain Organs. As a rule, Damp Heat retains the condition except for a pattern of Cold Damp in the Liver. Susceptible Organs are

Liver, Gallbladder and Spleen. Acupuncture makes use of needling to correct the states of Dampness, Hot or Cold.

(See Cirrhosis, Hepatitis)

Jaw and TMJ

The joint connecting the mandible or jawbone to the bone at the temple has a long name, the temporomandibular joint (TMJ), and that's a mouth full. This joint can be afflicted with injury, dislocation, stiffness, and arthritis. We hear the expression lockjaw, which differs as a symptom of tetanus.

No matter the source, two acupuncture points situated on both sides of the face relax the TMJ. Almost any associated disorder will benefit from these and other specific supplemental points. The outcome shows relaxation and comfortable jaw motion.

Knee Pain

A standard knee examination will search for evidence of injury, arthritic changes, and bursitis called housemaid's knee, excess joint fluid, and decreased mobility. Rheumatoid arthritis may show nodules and swellings. Medication by mouth or by injection gives relief. Additional forms of treatment incorporate physical therapy or surgery.

Chinese medicine's interpretations of knee disorders enter various categories. Injury with pain reflects Blockage of Circulation. The practitioner must know the Meridians involved and the type of Blockage—Hot, Cold, Damp, Congealed Blood. Recovery remains a matter of draining Obstructions and restoring Blood with the nutrients to heal damaged tissue.

Invasions of Wind, Damp, Cold or Heat produce arthritic changes.

The appearance of swelling and muscle degeneration labels this as crane's knee. Treatment releases the pathogenic invasions and strengthens bone by way of Kidney Qi.

Knee pain and weakness relate to Decreased Inherited Qi, or Essence, stored in the Kidney. Initially back and knee pains become noticed. You cannot replace the Qi but you can nourish it, strengthen it and vitalize it with acupuncture, moxa heat, and herbal remedies.

Acupuncture works through the Kidney to achieve maximum benefit. Furthermore, helpful acupuncture points for all knee problems are found on the leg, around the knee, back, ear, and scalp.

(See Arthritis)

Chapter 9
Laryngitis to Nose Problems

Laryngitis

Congestion and inflammation of the larynx leads to hoarseness or eventual voice loss. Causes include viruses or bacteria, and overuse of speech. Antibiotics and resting the vocal cords are therapeutic.

Lung Qi passes through the throat and governs the voice. Acupuncture will care for different complaints, depending on symptoms. A dry, raspy throat, for instance, requires lubrication and congestion calls for drainage.

The unique feature of laryngitis is voice disturbance. Since the Heart controls speech, it should be included in the treatment plan. This is an example of Chinese medicine's consideration of the body as a whole.

(See Voice Loss)

Leg Dysfunction

Many long Meridians travel the legs to and from the feet. Disorders can originate locally in the circulation or systemically out of Source Organs, or both. Needle stimulation in the lower extremity affects the upper regions. A point below the knee aids the Stomach and a point behind the knee relieves low back pain. Consequently, points near and far will strengthen the legs.

(See Knee Pain, Muscle Cramps, and Paralysis)

Leukemia

In leukemia, white blood cells reproduce in large numbers without restraint. They flow in the blood stream and infiltrate into some organs and tissues. The cells arise from the bone marrow. Some viruses are associated with the disease, but the true cause remains largely unknown. Chemotherapy, radiation and bone marrow transplant offer forms of treatment.

Acupuncture has taken its knowledge of dysfunctional bone marrow and formulated treatments. Kidney energy governs bone and produces marrow. Heart Qi controls Blood and the Spleen specifically manages Blood volume. All these components have a place in the therapeutic plan. Recommended also is a point that acts as the center of Bone Marrow. Reports from Asia indicate degrees of success using moxa heat. Several herbal combinations can help the condition as well.

Lyme Disease

A deer tick transmits a pathogen that may initially result in a skin lesion, followed by symptoms that may be flu-like, including fatigue, diarrhea, headache, stiff neck, chills and fever, followed by muscle and joint pain. Antibiotics are prescribed. If untreated, heart and nerve disorders may develop.

European history describes similar outbreaks; however, currently acupuncture usage has been limited. I have been able to relieve joint stiffness, yet one patient reacted with increased swelling. I believe that in time, accurate and designated Lyme Disease points will be established.

(See Infection)

Mania

Extreme excitability with aggressiveness describes the mental state of mania. This can shift to depression. Previously called manic-depressive illness, it is now known as bipolar mood disorder. There are subdivisions based on patient behavior and symptoms.

Acupuncture attributes the hostile personality to Phlegm Heat that agitates the Heart. Epilepsy and stroke are part of the same pattern. Cooling the Heat and expelling the Phlegm reverses the course of the disease. A needle prick technique bleeds and drains out Heat.

(See Emotions)

Mastitis

Inflammation and swelling of the breast occurs during breast-feeding from infection or cystic formation. There are no points on the breast for needling. Acupuncture, instead, works at a distance and around the mammary gland, while the patient wears a bra. Usually a favorable, immediate response provides relief. A few follow-up visits to complete or reinforce the correction may be deemed necessary.

Meniere's Disease

Symptoms include dizziness, gradual deafness, ringing and pressure in the ear. Uncertainties about the origin persist and conventional treatments use drugs and surgery.

Chinese medicine recognizes the cause in terms of Rising Liver Yang. The ascending Yang consists of a Heated force from the Liver that moves to the head as a troublemaker. Various happenings initiate the disease process such as the negative emotions of anger or depression, and lowered Cooling Yin. In turn, acupuncture anchors the Liver Yang and extinguishes the excess Liver Fire.

(See Deafness, Tinnitus)

Meningitis

Bacteria or viruses cause infection and inflammation of the spinal cord or brain membranes. The infection could come about from a remote source or from a concurrent disease. At times, infants and children are susceptible. This serious condition requires immediate attention to subdue the infection and relieve symptoms.

Heat invasion, a persistent Heat condition or weak immunity, describe the Chinese conception of causative factors. Most often, afflictions emanate in the seasons of spring and autumn. In some years, male college students become prone to the disease during spring, for which I devised a theory. Principles of Chinese medicine call attention to remnants of winter that remain even after the cold, wintry period has passed. These leftover chills pose a threat. Invasions enter the human body at the base of the skull into acupuncture points named Pools of Wind. The slightest touch of the seasonal change to warmth brings forth the desire in men to remove their shirts. Left unprotected, Wind blows in through the back of the neck and settles within the spine.

Acupuncture treatment clears Channels in the head and along the spine, and builds up immunity as well.

(See Infection)

Menopause

Due to natural hormonal changes beginning in a woman's forties, fifties, and sometimes thirties, the menstrual period will become irregular and finally stop. It is the time of menopause. This natural change can pass without discomfort. However, symptoms often appear as hot flashes, cold flashes, weakness, insomnia, lack of concentration, anger, and depressed feelings. Replacement of the hormone estrogen reduces the hot flushes and prevents osteoporosis (decreased bone density). The use of estrogen replacement therapy has been controversial.

Menopausal syndrome is a Chinese term identifying symptoms. To understand the energy workings that cause and cure these symptoms, we must look at the involved Channels and Organs. Two Channels take a major role in menstruation, the Penetrating and the Conception. The Penetrating Channel holds a supply of Blood in reserve. The Conception Channel controls the uterus and, if present, a fetus. The all-powerful force behind every function of reproduction lies with the Kidney.

Menopause occurs when the Penetrating Channel becomes deficient in Blood, the Conception Channel in control, and the Kidney in Qi. Kidney insufficiencies can lean either toward less Yin Qi or less Yang Qi. Symptoms depend on this shift.

The basis for types of discomfort derives from the phenomenon of Yin-Yang imbalances. Throughout life, women in general experience cool or chilly sensations. They are Yin. Men in contrast usually feel warmer, since they are Yang. Changes emanate during middle age of a male. By a seesaw effect, reduced Yin produces an empty form of Hot Yang; likewise, when Yang goes down Cold Yin ascends.

Most menopausal problems result from lowered cool Yin with rising hot Yang. Resultant symptoms consist of hot flashes, afternoon fevers, hot hands and feet, heart palpitations, insomnia, and night sweats. In the same realm of change, Kidney Yin Deficiency may induce Liver Yin Deficiency with issues of dizziness, blurry vision, and irritability. The less common Kidney Yang Deficiency brings about cold flashes, and bone changes.

Acupuncture attempts to reverse the uncomfortable sensations. When excess Heat dominates, it invigorates the Cool Yin and thus puts out the Fire. In all cases, treatment must regulate the Kidney, Liver, and related Channels. Herbal combinations also bring corrective relief.

Mental Disease

Mental function and dysfunction, intelligence, and the mind, all connect to the Brain. Yet acupuncture says we think with our Heart. Does Chinese medicine recognize a brain? Of course it does. The Brain serves as a miscellaneous Organ that works closely with Kidney Essence. Memory, concentration, hearing, and vision use the matter-of-fact Brain but led by the feelings of the Heart. Through the Heart, emotional and mental illnesses are improved.

Points of energy on the head connect to the Brain to treat injury, memory, attention deficit disorder, and retarded development. The Brain and Heart work well together.

Migraine Headache

Both Western and Chinese medicine classify types of headache according to areas of discomfort and related symptoms. Migraine falls into a unique classification. Sufferers generally see sparks or streaks of light before their eyes and endure digestive problems of nausea and vomiting. Pain frequently hits the forehead and temples. To Western medicine, causes can be hormonal, dietary, allergic, psychological, or the dilation of certain vessels. Family tendencies as described in the patient history have importance in evaluation.

Chinese medicine has identified the exact disease process. Unlike Western medicine, a headache is not a diagnosis in itself; instead it is one of several symptoms in a pattern of dysfunctional energy. Liver Fire Rising or Liver Yang Ascending sets off the complaint of migraine. These Syndromes show Hot Liver Qi going up to the head, which can occur with dizziness, high blood pressure, ringing in the ear, eye problems, and anger. Remember, whether in health or disease, Liver energy opens through the eyes.

Liver Qi strongly contributes to the energy of Stomach and Spleen, ruler of digestion. In the Cycle of Organs, Liver normally regulates Stomach and Spleen, but with excesses, they disrupt one another. Involvement of Stomach, Spleen, and the Liver-eye bond, explains the symptoms.

Acupuncture treatment strengthens the Liver, Stomach and Spleen. Any abundance is dispersed and local points around the eye are needled as needed.

Other headaches according to Western principles relate to

ailments such as sinus, ear, nose, and throat congestion. In addition, infections, injuries, poisons, fevers, emotional issues, and diseases of glands and organs contribute to the discomfort.

Acupuncture considers the sources of invasions and disharmonies to internal Organs. Wind-Cold, Wind-Heat or Wind-Dampness enters the head and Channels that bring forth a headache. The location of pain in the head and associated symptoms, point to the particular, affected Meridian. By clearing the area, correction takes place. Resultant Stagnation of Blood and Qi complicates a long-standing condition. In these cases, weather conditions such as rain, aggravate the existing trouble.

Organs have their place. Headache with heaviness, due to Stagnant Phlegm, comes about from Weak Spleen. A responsibility of Spleen resolves Dampness, so its repair cures the ailment. Combinations from external detrimental forces, with internal Organ Deficiency, require therapy in both regions.

As seen, the sources that foster headache symptoms are wide and varied. It involves much more than just a general ailment. Acupuncture thus recognizes and treats the complexities and problems of involved energy networks.

Multiple Sclerosis

The sheath that surrounds the spinal cord and brain breaks down in patches. The sheath is made of a substance called myelin and the disease process is called demyelination. Nerve weakness follows, which limits activities of limbs and vision. Various causes have been proposed such as viral infection, immune disorder, toxins, nutrient deficiencies, and a possible genetic component.

Multiple sclerosis in Chinese medicine is grouped under a heading of Atrophy Syndrome. This Syndrome contains diseases

133

of the disabled with impaired voluntary movements of leg and arm muscles. It seems that a condition of fever precedes the onset. Heat and Damp-Heat usually stay within the patient's energy system. Much attention goes to the Governing Vessel that parallels the spinal cord and penetrates the brain. As needed, Blockages along the Governing Vessel and Channels in regions of disability receive acupuncture to restore healthier Circulation. The Heat factor, if present, requires a cooling.

The sooner the patient gets treatment after diagnosis the better; the more delayed, the more limited the results. A school principal was referred to me after being diagnosed with multiple sclerosis. Internal Heat was very prevalent with back pain and stiff neck. Initial therapy cleared Heat and relieved the back and neck. Since then, he has come for acupuncture about every three months for nine years. Busy with his administrative work, he has had no setbacks. Now, the periodic visits care for minor symptoms.

(See Paralysis)

Muscle Cramps

Overuse of muscles may result in a cramp. This discomfort basically results from a contraction of muscle fibers. It could be occupational as in writer's cramp. Commonly, the calf muscle behind the leg suffers. Heat, massage, calcium or quinine by mouth and, believe it or not, the placement of a bar of soap on the leg, have been recommended.

In acupuncture, Liver governs muscle and maintains circulatory flow of Blood and Qi. Cramps in the calf very likely stem from Deficient Liver Blood. Often in the elderly, the cramps may include numbness and severe pain from related conditions of Stasis of Liver

Blood or complications of Wind and Phlegm. A needled acupuncture point at the muscle seems to give relief.

Muscular Dystrophy

Much research has taken place in this inherited disease, of which several forms are recognized. Although not a cure, acupuncture helps to strengthen by regulating the Inherited Qi in the Kidney and invigorating muscle energy.

Myasthenia Gravis

A mild-to-severe muscle weakness without atrophy, it affects the face, neck, spine, legs, and arms. A dysfunctional chemical exchange at the nerve muscle junction initiates the problem. Drug therapy restores nerve activity. Acupuncture placement harmonizes energy and invigorates spinal nerves, which may be of help.

Nausea

The unpleasant feeling of nausea that often leads to vomiting could be associated with early pregnancy (morning sickness), travel (seasickness, car sickness and airsickness), toxins, food poisoning, ill effects from drugs, repulsive odors, and disturbances of the nervous system or of the emotions. Nausea may also be present in digestive disorders related to the liver and gallbladder. Dizziness and headaches can accompany the queasiness. Medications called anti-emetic drugs suppress the nauseous sensation in various ways.

Stomach energy in Chinese medicine normally descends. However, certain disorders compel it to rise and induce nausea and sometimes vomiting. Rebellious Stomach Qi as this is called, frequently results from Damp Heat, which also provides an environment for infection. Damp Heat can occur in the Spleen, Liver, and Gallbladder. Stagnant or Deficient Stomach Qi and Stagnant Liver Qi produce nausea as well as some Cold disorders.

Morning sickness, resulting from pregnancy, is a different category and relates to a Channel that previously stored menstrual Blood, the Penetrating Channel. During pregnancy, an abundance of Qi remains here. Stomach Qi controls this Channel, whose excess in turn backs up and provokes the controlling Stomach Qi to rebel. Nausea can range from a mild—hardly noticeable—sensation to a severe outcome. Acupuncture regulates all these states of nausea by regulating the core Organ and sickness producing element.

Neck

Many structures make up the neck, joined intricately to the head and shoulders. Examination of spinal nerves, muscles, ligaments, and blood vessels assesses problems by physical range of motion, X-rays, and scans. Dysfunction appears perhaps due to injury, such as whiplash, poor posture, inflammation, infection, tumors, and bone degeneration.

I remember my first year in practice when I rented an office in a medical building. One day a man walked in with a complaint of neck pain. Searching for relief, he went from doctor to doctor. The best advice given was for a hot towel compress and pain medication. I had little more to offer. Oh, if I knew then what I know now.

While Western medicine studied anatomy of the neck, acupuncturists grew to understand the penetrating energy. Since Kidney Qi governs bone, its Deficiency lowers resistance. Then, arthritic changes easily take place. Liver dysfunction stiffens the neck from Stagnant Liver Qi or Hyperactive Liver Yang. Gallbladder Meridians travel the neck with other Channels.

Injury obstructs Blood and Qi circulation. It's important to identify the Channel involved. A common event describes Wind Cold Invasion, which causes a stiff neck. If complicated by a preexisting condition, this could lead to chronic neck pain. Heat and Damp also can invade. Depending on the diagnosis, acupuncture attempts to strengthen the Kidney, activate Stagnant Liver, decongest Channels and replenish with fresh Blood.

Effective therapeutic needling often is applied at a distance, such as the foot, ankle, wrist and hand. Healing points also exist in surrounding neck areas.

Nephritis

Nephritis means inflammation of the kidney caused by infection or toxins. It is often accompanied by fever. Diagnosis depends on urinalysis, bacterial cultures, scans and biopsies.

Acupuncture focuses on the pathogenic internal environment of Heat. Begun likely from a Wind-Heat invasion that drops through compartments of the body referred to as Upper, Middle and Lower Burners. Of course, the Heat yields fever and when in the Middle Burner, which contains Spleen and Stomach, digestive symptoms could arise. As it settles down into the Lower Burner, inflammation forms in the Kidney and Urinary Bladder. Swelling may result, sometimes of the eyelids.

Needling procedures reduce fever and clear Heat from the Lower Burner. If present, it also treats swelling in any part of the body.

Nerve Diseases

Acupuncture treats all types of nerve diseases, e.g., those of abnormal sensation or those of impaired movement. Remarkably, nerves, as structures that transfer impulses have no place in Traditional Chinese Medicine. Energy takes responsibility for all activities Western medicine attributes to nerve function. Many think of acupuncture as affecting nerves. Actually, acupuncture influences all body parts, organs, muscles, arteries, and notwithstanding, nerves. But we are not performing nerve blocks for pain. I looked up the Chinese word for nerve in my Chinese Medical Dictionary and found none.

Although there is some correspondence, in that certain Channels run parallel along, and influence the spine to benefit disability. However, it is best not to confuse nerves with the circulation of energy.

Nose Problems

Problems of the nose include nosebleed, rhinitis, inflammation of the nostril lining associated with sinus congestion or allergies, polyp formation, loss of the sense of smell (anosmia), swelling, and pain. The protruding location on the face makes it susceptible to injury. For hemorrhage, application of pressure at the bridge of the nose or nostrils has long been an emergency measure for control. Specific acupuncture points can also stop the bleeding.

In Chinese medicine, Lung Qi opens at the nose. This means that invasions of pathogenic elements (Cold, Heat, Dry and Heat) with Wind in the Lungs, will effect disorders of the nose accordingly, with white, yellow, light or heavy discharge. Clearing congestion and obstruction in the nostrils, and regulating the Lungs, improves breathing, opens sinuses, shrinks polyps and restores a sense of smell. Of course, response varies from person to person.

A swollen red nose indicates Heat, thrown off by the Stomach, Spleen, Heart, Liver, or Lung. Pain, however, results from Wind Invasion, Heat, Dampness, or Stagnant Blood Circulation.

(See Allergy, Common Cold)

Chapter 10
Pain to Stroke

Pain

Western medicine regards pain as a symptom related to a disorder. Well, so does acupuncture. The difference stands out in Western medicine's emphasis on disturbances to nerve-ending receptors due to inflammation, infection, injury, or pressure. Location of the distress in both health professions has importance to uncover the source of distress. Diagnosis depends on identifying abnormal structures, pathological changes, and faults in body chemistry.

Chinese medicine analyzes the nature and qualities of pain and what aggravates or alleviates it. The disease-causing element bears directly on treatment. Rather than cells, tissues, and biochemistry, discomfort is diagnosed and remedied within the body's energy system.

The patient-doctor consultation discloses a lot of information. Do certain weather conditions make the problem worse? This serves as a diagnostic question. For example, if the problem feels better with heat, it is a Cold condition. Inquiries search for Deficiency, Excess, Stagnancy, Congealed Blood, and Dampness. Once the abnormal Qi cause of pain becomes established, its manner of elimination accurately corresponds to the problem. Acupuncture precisely removes Excess Cold, Stagnation, and Dampness.

Palpitation

Rapid or irregular beating of the heart is called palpitation. ECG (electrocardiogram) examination searches for defects in conductivity. Chinese medicine attributes the problem to Heart Deficiencies of Qi, Blood, Yin, or Yang. Frequently, too much Heat in the Heart activates the fluttering from Deficient Heart Yin. An exact assessment is put together with other symptoms, such as shortness of breath, insomnia, dizziness, forgetfulness, and lethargy. Acupuncture regulates the Organ. Also, Kidney Qi warrants attention, since it is responsible for Heart balance.

(See Heart Problems)

Paralysis

The loss of motor function or sensation in a body part indicates paralysis. Caused by a lesion or damage to nerve cells (neurons), muscle tone and voluntary movement diminish. Psychology has described hysterical paralysis, without the location of a lesion.

Spinal injuries receive traction and immobilization to prevent additional trauma. Rehabilitative physical therapy and emotional support can assist.

Interference of Qi and Blood flow, through major Channels, is a matter of great concern in acupuncture. Those that enter the Brain and spinal column must be needled to invigorate fresh Circulation.

I have observed in my office how scalp acupuncture, which directly energizes the Brain, has proven to be a wonderful supplement in rehabilitation. Depending on the patient's condition, miracles do seem to happen.

Parkinson's Disease

This progressive neurological disorder results in stooped posture, shuffling gait, slow and weak movement, muscle stiffness, and tremor at rest. Characteristic of Parkinson's is a rolling motion of the hand and fingers. Degeneration occurs in a part of the brain that controls movement. The average age of onset is 60. Various drugs inhibit some loss of control.

Chinese medicine recognizes a disease process of Internal Wind from the Liver. This must not be confused with External Wind invasion that produces chills, fever, coughs, and respiratory illness that may lead to a digestive problem. Instead, stirring activities take place within the body. Evidence of Wind displays moving and shaking, signs of Parkinson's.

Liver Wind comes about by Deficient Liver Blood. An important Liver function stores Blood, which nourishes tendons and possibly nerves. The cool-stable Liver Yin, when Deficient, can become a rising Liver Yang and then Wind. Extreme Heat also injures the Liver Meridian and energy levels that result in Wind.

Acupuncture therapy suppresses the internal Wind by replenishing the Liver Blood supply. Enhancement of Qi will restore Blood. Then stronger Yin will anchor the uncontrolled rising Yang. Drainage of excess Heat as indicated greatly helps. Brain points on the head offer additional means of recovery.

Pediatric Diseases

Childhood (pediatric) diseases generally respond well to acupuncture. In my experience, compared to adults, fewer needles and shorter treatment periods achieve correction. It behooves a practitioner to remember that growth continues even during an affliction. For instance, the stomach grows and digests at the same time. A helpful made-for-young-age needle application on the hand easily remedies the child's digestive system.

Usually, children accept acupuncture. They find the healing process a pleasant experience. I use smaller, thinner needles and often, just massage and pressure will suffice.

The controversial subject of immunization should be addressed. Years before Edward Jenner discovered inoculation for smallpox in the late eighteenth century, a doctor in China made similar findings. Today, routine vaccination builds a child's immunity against several diseases. Parents are divided between acceptance and rejection of this practice. Many choose no vaccines, except for polio.

Chinese medical principles give a different insight. Acupuncture effectively treats mumps, chicken pox, and whooping cough. If accessible, no need exists for the vaccine. Measles is placed in a unique category. Poisons from birth remain within the child until an episode of measles releases them, during which acupuncture can relieve symptoms. Toxic retention could cause future disorders. As in adult illnesses, Chinese medicine has individual interpretations. Mumps, for example, results from an accumulation of Wind, Damp, and Heat around the jaw, treatable by acupuncture.

Pelvic Inflammatory Disease

During my internship years in the hospital emergency room, women

143

with painful pelvic inflammatory disease (PID) were common walk-ins. Basically an infection of the fallopian tubes, PID may include the cervix, uterus, and ovaries. It is sexually transmitted, abetted possibly by birth-control devices (IUDs). Treatment consists of identification and elimination of pathogens.

Acupuncture puts the symptoms together with the patient's description of any vaginal discharge to make the diagnosis. With disease-making conditions in mind, there is differentiation of Damp Heat and Stagnation of Blood, or Liver Qi. The Liver Channel encircles reproductive organs. Stagnation of Cold within this Vessel also produces the disease. Each unhealthy type of internal environment directly undergoes therapy, by acupuncture or herbs, to restore normal function. Consequently, the infection disappears.

(See Infection)

Pneumonia

Lung inflammation mainly from bacteria, viruses, or irritating substances defines pneumonia. It can develop as a complication of other diseases. Antibiotics and supportive care are the treatments of choice. Vaccination for a common bacterial cause of pneumonia is available as well as for influenza. However, pneumonia continues to be a frequent reason for hospital death.

This Lung affliction, in Chinese medicine, denotes Heat and Dryness. A Wind Heat has invaded to effect symptoms of fever, thirst, sore throat, dry cough, and constipation. To reverse the sickness, Wind and Heat must leave the body, as the Lungs decongest and cool down.

Acupuncture commentary on Western medicine, explains that antibiotics such as penicillin provide a cooling or Yin boosting property in addition to antibacterial action. Secondly, excessive blood letting from the inner elbow veins for laboratory tests, overlap a Lung Meridian. This could weaken the Lungs.

(See Infection)

Post-traumatic Stress Disorder (PTSD)

More severe than stress or fear, posttraumatic stress disorder bursts forth after a terrifying event, ordeal, or life-threatening experience such as in military combat, natural disasters, and accidents. The person relives the encounter with frightening thoughts and emotional upset.

Since Chinese medicine never separated the body from the emotions, and treats both through needle stimulation, acupuncture offers a great deal of help for stress disorders. Patients relax and allow the healing to take place.

Thousands of research years resulted in many methods to improve the psyche. Head parts, Organs, and Channels all come into use. Scalp acupuncture energizes the Brain with increased strength. Regarded as an extension of the Brain, the ear reflects the entire body. Certain auricular points enhance emotions and normalize the autonomic nervous system. The emotional Heart is stimulated directly. And needled Channels that connect one another will add power.

A woman suffered terrible psychological trauma from an automobile accident.

She saw me because she constantly recalled the agonizing episode. She experienced panic attacks and physical pain. I applied every compatible needle combination I knew to help her and she responded well.

(See Emotions)

Premenstrual Syndrome (PMS)

Approximately seven to ten days before menstruation, negative emotions such as depression, distress, or uneasiness, appear accompanied by headaches, bloating, or breast pain. It lasts until the menses begin. These symptoms comprise PMS, which Western medicine attributes to hormonal imbalance.

Specific symptoms achieve relief with indicated treatment. Hormone therapy regulates estrogen and progesterone, counseling and antidepressants aid the emotions, diuretics reduce swelling and bloating.

Chinese medicine lists the same symptoms but relates them to Organ energy imbalances, mostly of the Liver that stores Uterine Blood. Stagnant Liver Qi brings on depression and irritability as well as swollen breasts. It ascends and headaches develop. Extreme Heat in both Liver and Heart projects feelings of Fire as anger and agitation. A large number of PMS discomforts relate to Organ disharmonies corrected by acupuncture.

Prolapse of Uterus and Rectum

Prolapse refers to a body structure that drops down. This condition is most often seen with the uterus and rectum. Procedures use non-invasive support or surgical repair, leaning more toward conservative taping methods for children with rectal prolapse. In older adults, the annoyance turns up as a complication from severe hemorrhoids.

Through applied knowledge of Chinese medical science, prolapsed structures return to their proper place. We find the answers in

Spleen Qi. As with every Organ energy, Spleen energy performs a number of tasks. One upholds Organs and tissues in their position. When Spleen Qi Sinks or suffers Deficiency, problems of prolapse befall. To correct, Spleen Qi receives the needed strength to power elevation and provide holding stability. In addition, the weakened area directly has treatment. One point to uplift energy throughout the body is located on top of the head.

For office treatment of prolapsed uterus, I tell the patient to push back the protrusion by hand. While on her side, acupuncture is administered. Maintained support usually follows, but reinforcement often becomes necessary.

(See Hemorrhoids)

Prostate Problems

The prostate secretes fluid to transport sperm for reproduction. Found beneath the bladder, and wrapping around the urethra (the canal to transport urine or semen in males), it enlarges as a man ages. Frequent urination and diminished flow result.

Three common prostate ailments are inflammation or prostatitis, non-cancerous enlargement called benign prostatic hypertrophy, and prostate cancer. Digital or ultrasound examinations evaluate the size and structure of the gland. Biopsy may also be performed.

Indicated treatments include antibiotics for prostatitis, resection through the urinary passage for enlargement, and radiation, hormonal therapy, or complete surgical removal in cases of cancer. In the case of cancer, medical opinions vary as to monitoring or removal.

In acupuncture procedures, emphasis is placed on the urinary symptoms with the associated tongue and pulse examination. Pathological conditions in the genital-prostate region require an assessment and a treatment strategy to restore normalcy. Frequent patterns involve Damp-Heat, Damp-Cold, Kidney Deficiency, and Stagnant Qi or Blood.

Different needle combinations apply to each syndrome. Through the rehabilitation of the internal environment, urinary function and prostate structure improve. Specific prostate acupuncture leg points are found by palpation for tenderness.

In general, treatment regulates the Kidney and works on the Conception Vessel. This Channel passes through the body's midline and related Organs in the lower abdomen. The Spleen provides additional help by reducing swelling and invigorating circulation; the Liver activates Stagnation. Also, the Liver Meridian deserves attention, since it completely encircles the genitalia.

The same needle formula that treats prostate problems also prevents them. Effective in the early stages, it is best to begin when the urinary annoyances are minor.

Psoriasis

The most common form of this skin disease is called plaque, characterized by silvery scaling on raised, reddish lesions that are commonly seen on the scalp, elbows, knees, and lower back. Psoriasis may develop elsewhere on the body. It is generally recognized as an autoimmune disease with a genetic component. Patients frequently find help by the application of lubricating medication on the skin, phototherapy (exposure to sunlight or lamplight), drug therapy, water therapy, diet, and now, alternative medicine.

Chinese medicine interprets the problem in its own way. Dryness has significance. Deficiencies in energy levels deep below the outer surface create a condition that allows Wind invasions. They combine with elements of Hot or Cold and maybe Damp. Eventually, it all changes to Heat, and Heat with Wind produces Dryness. Prolonged negative emotions may produce Heat as well. The general outcome is Stagnant Qi and Blood. This encourages lesion formation.

Close observation of the skin reveals details of underlying origins. In addition to silver for example, a whitish hue is a hint of Cold; red with slight greasiness may mean Damp Heat; dark spots of color indicate Stagnation.

Treatment directly cares for the condition. Included are standard acupuncture points for all cases of dermatology, which adjust Blood and Qi. I always supplement acupuncture with oral herbal remedies, indicated for the disharmony.

Ten to 30% of patients with psoriasis will develop psoriatic arthritis. I have not come across much information on this entity in Chinese medicine. Since disturbances of Blood circulation are a causative factor for both, I think it should serve as the basis for assessment and treatment.

(See Arthritis)

Purpura (Purple Patches)

Not a common disease, but since it has long been seen in China with acupuncture diagnosis and treatment, purpura is included here. The disorder involves blood forced out of the vessels into the skin and mucous membranes leaving a recognizable purple patch that does not blanch when pressed.

Besides the skin, the bleeding condition can affect the stomach, intestines and joints. Severity differs among patients. Primarily a childhood disease, but adults are not exempt. It frequently follows a bacterial infection or at times a drug reaction, but is usually due to platelet disorders. Steroids are customarily used to treat the problem.

Chinese medicine describes two separate courses of development for the disease. An abundance of Heat in the Blood forces hemorrhage to occur. The other process results from Deficient Spleen Qi. The Spleen produces, manages and upholds Blood flow. Depending on the evaluation, the application of acupuncture either eliminates the Heat or invigorates the Spleen.

Reflux

Reflux refers to a backward flow. In connection with the stomach it means regurgitation up into the esophagus, due to dysfunction of the sphincter muscle between the esophagus and stomach. Called gastroesophageal reflux disease (GERD), over time if untreated, ulcers and other tissue changes may occur in the esophagus. Reflux does not always take place after eating; instead, it could act up at strange times such as the next day or late in the night. The principal symptom is heartburn, treated with a modified diet and antacids.

Acupuncture evaluates the symptoms that accompany reflux to determine the pathogenic condition in the Stomach. Among the disease producers are Cold, Stagnation, Damp-Heat, Food Retention, Blood Stasis, and Deficiencies of Yin or Qi. A Sour Regurgitation results in certain situations, for instance if Liver Qi invades the Stomach.

Correction progresses as harmful substances drain off and the self-regulating Organ Qi goes to work. For convenience, the acupuncturist and patient can make an appointment to administer needling, before, during or after an episode.

(See Gastritis, Indigestion)

Rheumatic Disease

The medical science or specialty that works with rheumatic disease is called rheumatology. Rheumatologists study and treat disorders of joints, connective tissue, and soft tissues. Common characteristics of these diseases exhibit inflammation, stiffness, joint pain, and swelling.

Diagnosis and treatment for rheumatoid arthritis is complicated and made by physical examination, laboratory studies, cytology (study of cells), and X-rays. Treatment employs analgesics, steroids, and physiotherapy. The various medications are taken orally, by injection, or both.

A different attitude toward the disease in Traditional Chinese Medicine stems from ancient concepts. Rheumatic disease does not directly translate into Chinese. Whereas tissue and chemical changes due to inflammation carries much importance in Western medicine, significance in China's medicine comes from the type of pain. Acupuncture interprets Blockage pain, known as Bi pain, derived from invasions of Wind, Cold, Dampness or Heat. Questioning reveals painful Obstructions of Excess, Deficiency, Stagnation, and others. This information serves as a basis for diagnosis and treatment. Acupuncture and herbal formulas provide many benefits to reduce Heat, regenerate Joints and restore Blood and Qi circulation.

(See Arthritis)

Rheumatic Fever

Rheumatic fever primarily afflicts youngsters between 5 and 15 years of age. It begins as a feverish infectious disease of childhood, caused by a bacteria called Group A streptococcus, which can affect the heart, joints, skin, and brain. The anti-inflammatory actions of aspirin and antibiotics established a standard form of treatment. If untreated, damage to the heart valves will usually develop.

Chinese medicine places rheumatic fever in the same pattern of Blockage as rheumatoid arthritis and connective tissue diseases. The fever develops from Accumulation of Damp Heat that obstructs Channels. Acupuncture applications and herbal formulas address the syndrome. Treatment reduces fever and clears Channels of Damp Heat.

Sciatica

Sciatica refers to pain along the sciatic nerve, the large nerve that runs down the lower back, through the buttocks, thighs, and legs. One can experience severe discomfort or disability within these areas if the nerve is compressed or irritated. Pain may fluctuate or stay constant.

Physical therapy treatment depends on the underlying cause and routinely uses knee and hip flexion exercises. Chiropractic performs adjustments and medical practitioners prescribe analgesics (painkillers) and muscle relaxants. Surgical correction may be required for a herniated disc.

In Chinese medicine, sciatica symptoms are due to Kidney Qi Deficiency, since Kidney governs the skeletal system, or Painful Obstruction in a Channel, which identifies a state of Excess. Enhancing the Kidney helps the Deficiency difficulty. However, the exact Channel and type of Blockage corresponds to selected acupuncture application. Regularly, the Gallbladder and Urinary Bladder Channels clog up and the Blockage itself may consist of Blood Stagnation, Wind, Cold, or Dampness.

Needling clears the Obstruction and normalizes Blood and Qi

circulation. Over the centuries, acupuncture has formulated specific and effective points. A good supplement uses areas on the ear.

Shingles

Inflammation and little blister-like formations on the skin signify shingles. Frequently occurring along the course of a nerve at the ribcage or waist; I recently treated a man on the head, down the neck and arm. Patients may experience extreme discomfort. The same virus that causes chickenpox infects nerve branches off the central nervous system. Steroids are often prescribed and there is now a vaccination to prevent shingles.

Acupuncture interprets a Toxic Wind Fire, which injures body fluids. The affected Channels are identified. Then dispersing the Wind and Fire with application to detoxify will remedy the disorder. I have found that a needling method under the lesion gives much relief and hastens the cure.

Shoulder Pain

Shoulder pain comes about from a variety of reasons. Three of the most common are bursitis, tendonitis, and a torn rotator cuff. This joint is unique in its range of motion; however limitations in elevating and rotating the arm frequently occur with painful injuries. I treat sports injuries in the fields of tennis, golf, crew, baseball, and football. Pain and stiffness result from invasions of Wind, Cold, and Dampness. The Cold induces contraction and constrained motion. Dampness can lead to swelling.

Patient care initially eliminates congestion. Often I employ the herbal heat of moxa (mugwort) to drive out the Cold and Dampness, as I activate fresh circulation. A Meridian network crosses the shoulder, transporting Organ energies. Corrective help uses Stomach, Large Intestine, Urinary Bladder, and Heart Qi. Progress is made as pain decreases and range of motion increases. Often sports activities are resumed during a course of therapy without further harm.

Sinus Congestion

A sinus refers to an open space or cavity usually in a bone. Frequently, sinuses around the nose become congested or infected. Physicians keep in mind sources of the infection from bacteria, viruses, or fungi. Another basis for the irritation ties to allergies and environmental influences. Antibiotics, decongestants, and nasal sprays are common treatments.

Acupuncture views the nose—including connected sinuses—as the external opening for the Lung. The ailment stems from Wind Heat or Damp Heat in the Lung, which also fosters infection. Needle application clears the Lung plus involved Channels beside, above and under sinuses. Correction occurs by removing Heat and draining congestion, even down to the foot.

(See Allergies, Infection)

Sleep Apnea

When breathing is interrupted during sleep, due to airway obstruction, it is called sleep apnea. This can occur many times throughout the night. If severe, apnea leads to high blood pressure, cardiovascular disease, memory problems, weight gain, and even death. Diagnosed usually by observations in sleep studies, treatment calls for lifestyle changes from poor habits. Decreasing alcohol consumption and smoking, using oral appliances, or a continuous positive airway pressure (CPAP) device, aid the condition. Extreme cases may require surgery where excess tissue is removed from the throat. Basically not serious, but with obesity and heart impairment there could be a vital situation of life or death. Airway obstruction shows a reason in mechanics for the breathless state.

Acupuncture recognizes the obstruction and works to clear the respiration. Needles concentrate on a major Channel that runs along the chest. Additional points promote general strength and regulate the Lungs. I stimulate a Kidney point in the lower abdomen that anchors the breath during a deep inhalation exercise.

Stroke (Cerebrovascular Accident or CVA)

Stroke occurs when the blood supply to the brain is interrupted due to a clot blocking a blood vessel, hemorrhage (bleeding), or abnormal blood vessel function. Risk factors include hypertension, advanced age, diabetes, smoking, and elevated cholesterol levels. Medically, also known as apoplexy, nursing care and rehabilitative exercises make up a treatment plan. In about half the cases, when not too severe, degrees of recovery prove possible.

Chinese medicine categorizes different types of stroke according to signs and symptoms. This classification aids in the selection of needle combinations. Prior to the understanding of changes in cerebral blood flow, acupuncture documented a pathological process. Other than injury, it reveals a deeper awareness of the disease.

The more we know about stroke, the better for all practices of medicine, since it is the second leading cause of death in the United States, and 75% of people suffering a stroke have significant disabilities.

During the initial emergency period, needling and moxa heat jointly attempt to resuscitate the afflicted. Well points at the distal

155

tips of the Channels and a spot on the head possibly are bled. The so-called Well points act as starting and finishing places for Qi and ideally serve for drainage of excesses that promote a stroke. They may also take an acupuncture needle in the acute stage. Moxa supports the Inherited Qi, the Essence (the reserve of life) at the navel.

Conditions following the attack, called the sequelae, often benefit from acupuncture. Disabilities of the lower and upper extremities undergo evaluation and rehabilitation. Other concerns include speech disorders and facial paralysis.

Overall, there are two general divisions: Channel stroke and Organ stroke. When limited to Channels, a less threatening mild stroke occurs, affecting extremities and torso. There is no loss of consciousness. But the dangerously serious Organ stroke puts the patient into a comatose state.

A further subdivision presents two additional sets of symptoms as "closed" and "open". The closed shows clenched fists and teeth, fever and red complexion. In contrast, the open has a relaxed mouth, relaxed hands and a pale complexion.

The Chinese name for stroke translates as Center Wind or Wind Stroke. Wind originates in the Liver and ascends though the Heart to the Brain. Then afterward comes a brain hemorrhage. In the same initial Syndrome we find high blood pressure and epilepsy. Another complicating factor that blocks the senses is Phlegm accumulation.

The sequence begins with prolonged negative emotions such as depression and frustration. This affects the Liver to produce rising Wind, which travels up through the Heart and into the Brain. Acupuncture treats accordingly.

(See Coma, Paralysis)

Chapter 11
Tennis Elbow to Weight Gain

Tennis Elbow

Pain at the outer side of the elbow joint indicates tennis elbow. It is where the tendons of the forearm muscles attach to the elbow and become inflamed. It is an overuse injury caused not only by playing tennis, but other common motions such as raking or painting. Similar strain to the to the arm's inner side is golfer's elbow, since golfers swing inward. Many categorize the joint pain as a bursitis. Treatments employ ice applications, physical therapy, analgesics, anti-inflammatory medication or a flexible brace.

Acupuncture sees the problem in terms of harm to the circulatory network in the arm. Deficiency and Stagnation of Qi and Blood result. Since Chinese medicine believes the body has the ability to heal from within, Qi and nutrients of Blood repair the damage. A blocked Blood flow, however, cannot reach the injured tissue. To correct, needling opens blockages, drains Stagnation and replenishes Qi and Blood.

In my experience, allowing the patient to heal offers the best outcome. As acupuncture improves the condition, followed by less pain and more mobility, people may search for a supplemental therapy, sometimes without informing the acupuncturist. This can happen in the midst of care for other types of trauma or disability.

A rule of thumb for additional treatment is gentleness. The progress made through acupuncture unfortunately can be undone with forceful manipulation or extreme muscle stretching. I recommend very light massage as an adjunct. Once acupuncture accomplishes substantial correction, more zealous therapy may be tried.

(See Bursitis)

Throat

The throat itself deserves attention. It provides the outlet for the Lung and houses the vocal cords. Almost every Channel passes through, which become involved with surrounding disorders and offers a means for their correction. Application of this knowledge cares for dry, parched or sore throat, hoarseness, loss of voice, hyperthyroidism, tonsillitis, and laryngitis.

(See Laryngitis, Hyperthyroidism, Goiter, Tonsillitis, Voice Loss)

Tinnitus (Ringing in the Ear)

Ringing, buzzing, hissing or other noises in the ear, that fluctuate or stay constant, diagnose tinnitus. It's subjective, meaning that only the patient hears the sound. Causes include loud noises, blockages, infections, foreign bodies, growths, injury, toxins, prescribed drugs, and systemic diseases. The disorder may lead to hearing loss.

Mechanical devices have been used for therapy; also pleasant music has masked the noise. The intensity of the condition varies among people.

Acupuncture groups related symptoms such as headache, dizziness, reduced appetite, and congested lungs, into specific syndromes. These involve Organ Deficiencies that fail to provide enough Qi and Blood, or Essence. Rising Liver Heat and Phlegm Stagnation are other pathologies. Treatment normalizes the disharmonies and directly opens the ear.

(See Deafness, Meniere's Disease)

Tiredness

Both Western and Chinese medicine agree that tiredness or fatigue results from exhaustion, deficiencies, viral or parasitic infections, and psychological problems. More specifically, our conventional medicine says it lies in the lack of nerve stimulation, physical organ dysfunction, metabolic waste buildup, and mental unevenness. Compare this to Organ Qi or Yang Deficiencies, heaviness from retained Dampness or Phlegm and Stagnancy due to negative emotions,

Acupuncture lists other symptoms alongside the fatigue to get to the Organ disharmony. For example, digestive disorders with poor appetite and abdominal pain, which is reduced from pressure applied by hand, explains Deficiency of the Large Intestine or Spleen Qi or Yang Deficiency. Correcting the Organ renews wakefulness and relieves the symptoms as well.

Tonsillitis

What Western medicine classifies as inflammation caused by

159

infection, Chinese medicine considers a condition of Damp or Phlegm in the enlarged tonsils. Instead of antibiotics and bed rest, or tonsillectomy, acupuncture clears out the involved Lung Channel by needling and opening the end point on the thumb.

The Chinese hospital where I received my acupuncture training treated about seven thousand patients a day. All conceivable health resources were made available: ICU (intensive care unit), obstetrics, American medicine, Chinese medicine, emergency medicine, and surgery. Thousands of people had acupuncture—both in the hospital wards and outpatient clinics. Thousands received Chinese massage therapy; thousands took herbal medication, orally and intravenously. Among the masses of sick, only two or three underwent surgery in a day. Many disorders that the West treats with surgical procedures, China uses acupuncture instead.

(See Infection)

Toothache

Energy Meridians pass in and around the mouth and jaws. Needles can drain congestion down to the foot and can regulate Blood circulation. Kidney Qi favorably acts upon bone and teeth. Many dental problems receive help with acupuncture, for example, abscess, inflammation of gums (gingivitis), and TMJ (temporomandibular joint) syndrome. Actually an acupuncture point under the cheekbone loosens the stiff jawbone joints.

Patients sometimes request me at their dentist's office. Before, during and after their procedure I administer acupuncture. In addition to relaxation, it reduces pain and aids in healing.

Also, I have hastened healing after corrective dental work. Points on the hand and foot are especially useful. A Channel begins under the eye, crosses the gums and jaws, and travels down to the foot. Needle regulation at distal areas will make improvement at the other end, in the mouth. A point on the hand helps anything in the head. Working on the network of energy Channels treats most ailments. This web is connected throughout the body. However, certain needled points along a line elicit certain responses.

(See Jaw, TMJ)

Trauma

Trauma refers to physical or emotional injury. In either case, acupuncture and energy systems apply. No matter what body structure or mental component becomes damaged, it also harms the integrated Qi. Therefore, treatment aims to correct the dimension of injured energy, which reverses the anatomical or psychological trauma.

A broken bone, for instance, may be immobilized in a cast or splint. In China, needles are inserted above and below the cast. I have done this in my office and observed quicker healing. Because acupuncture never separated the physical realm from one's feelings, the emotions receive therapy also by needling indicated points.

(See Emergencies, Emotions, Post-Traumatic Stress Disorder)

Trigeminal Neuralgia (Face Pain)

Two terms with the same meaning describe face pain—trigeminal neuralgia and tic douloureux. The severe discomfort relates to the trigeminal nerve, which has three main branches going to the upper part of the face and head, and upper and lower jaw. With an unknown cause, theories center on nerve compression, trauma, or infection.

Chinese medicine differentiates causes of Wind, Cold, and Heat invasions to the face, and prolonged negative emotions. Acupuncture needling eliminates the pathogenic factor or improves sensibilities. Sometimes, Channels are opened at a distance. Usually, pain diminishes at a slow but gradual pace.

(See Bell's Palsy)

Tuberculosis

Tuberculosis is a disease, which Western medicine ascribes to infection by an organism called Mycobacterium tuberculosis or the tubercle bacillus. Although usually found in the lung, this contagious disease can occur in various parts of the body, i.e., organs, glands, bones, and joints. Discoveries of human remains have shown its presence from thousands of years ago.

Treatment by Western standards includes long term antibiotic therapy, good diet, and in some cases, bed rest.

Chinese medicine evaluates a Syndrome of Deficient Lung Yin with fiery symptoms of dry mouth and coughing, possibly with blood, fever, and red complexion. Yin acts as the body's cooling and moisturizing power. Every Organ tries to maintain a stabilizing Yin-Yang balance. When the Yin drops as in this case, the Yang dominates and heats up the body. Of course, the unhealthy internal environment invites bacteria growth.

Acupuncture aims to Drain Excess Heat and restore Deficient Yin in the Lung, and in affiliated Organs chiefly the Kidney and Spleen. In other words, it cools things down and reverses symptoms. Quite often, Western medication and acupuncture needling compatibly work together in these types of cases.

Of interest, a designated pair of acupuncture points was historically developed for tuberculosis of the bone. Found to be the center of all bone energy, today it treats any disorder of the skeletal system.

(See Infection)

Ulcers

An ulcer appears as an open sore on the skin or mucous membrane. Inflammation or infection may also be present.

Injury, extreme heat or cold, and poor blood circulation will allow for tissue breakdown. Prolonged pressure at a bony prominence—knee, heel and buttock—after confinement to bed for a long period of time, often results in a bedsore called a decubitus ulcer. A cast can also ulcerate the skin. Diabetics are prone to foot ulcers due to weak blood flow. Cleansing, with protective bandaging of the wound, aids in repair.

Internally, ulcers occur in the mouth, on the tongue, in the esophagus, in the stomach (gastric ulcer), small intestine (peptic ulcer), and large intestine (ulcerative colitis). Western medicine often connects dietary deficiencies and infectious disease to changes in the mouth. Infection with bacteria, excess stomach acid, poor diet, and a stressful way of life, provoke ulcers in the digestive system. Treatment emphasizes antacids, antibiotics, and emotional support if necessary.

Chinese medicine interprets ulcers in the mouth and on the tongue as signs of Excess Heart Fire or Blazing Stomach Fire. Energy of the Heart opens to the tongue and from the Stomach, into the mouth. Acupuncture therapy in both Syndromes operates to "put out the fire", by dispersing the excess Yang Fire and enhancing the cooling Yin—all done through physiological reactions to needling.

Stomach ulcers fall into a category of a Cold condition. If accompanied by stabbing pain, it shows Congealed Blood. Related Syndromes involve the Stomach, Spleen or Small Intestine. Treatment is directed to disperse the Cold and then Warm the Organs. Some moxa herbal heat provides a good supplement.

Now in regards to ulcerated skin, a prescription of needled points improves surface circulation. In addition, stimulation near and around the ulcer promotes closure.

(See Foot Problems, Gastritis, Reflux)

Urinary Problems

Our conventional medicine lists a number of bladder ailments as separate entities with their own pathologies and treatments. These consist of increased or decreased urinary frequency, stones, urinary tract infection, and urogenital disorders that affect both the reproductive and urinary systems.

Laboratory assessments yield a wealth of information on kidney and bladder defects through findings of toxins, infection, and biochemical imbalances. X-ray, invasive and noninvasive instrument examinations (i.e., ultrasound), and biopsy add to the picture. Of course, we must not dismiss the importance of hereditary and congenital influences.

Depending on diagnostic data, available indicated treatment offers a wide range of choices, from dietary management, antibiotics, and surgical correction of defects, to dialysis and organ transplant for kidney failure.

The disorders actually represent symptoms of Chinese Syndromes. In depth understanding of the disease process explains the Syndrome. Deficiencies of Kidney Essence, Yang, or Bladder Qi, all lacking strength, permit incontinence. The big supporter, Spleen Qi, can Sink and lead to incontinence. Deficient Kidney Yin that results in too much Heat causes urogenital trouble. Kidney or Bladder stones form from Damp Heat, like dough baking to bread or clay hardening to earthenware. A urinary tract infection begins with Heat in the Heart, which drops into the Small Intestine. This Organ separates the pure and impure and makes urine. When Heat dominates, infection can follow.

Another Heart link recognized in Western and Eastern medicine pertains to Kidney failure with a weakened Heart. A connection suggests congestive heart failure as the kidney holds in fluid, resulting in decreased circulation to the organs to include the kidney. Reduced intake of salt and diuretics provide some needed patient care.

The traditional energy cycle shows how the Kidney, symbolized by Water, regulates the Heart, the Fire symbol. Water controls Fire. An impaired Kidney cannot manage the Heart. They both suffer. Accordingly, acupuncture repair of the Heart frequently incorporates the Kidney, especially for Yang and Yin imbalances.

(See Nephritis)

Vaginitis

As the name implies, vaginitis means inflammation and infection of the vagina. Douching may change the internal environment, allowing infection to develop. Administration of antibiotics for another condition, i.e., bronchitis, may eradicate the normal flora, causing overgrowth of yeast. Possible sources include bacteria, fungi, and irritants in douching. Practices of proper female hygiene in cleansing the area ought to render treatment and prevention.

Chinese assessments involve disease-producing Heat, i.e., Damp Heat, Heat from Deficient Yin, Heat in the Blood. Patient experience has more importance then an examination. A complete evaluation takes in symptoms as itching, burning discomfort, dryness or discharge. Specific needle applications will disperse Heat, cool down the pelvic region and lubricate the dryness.

Voice Loss

The Lung governs the voice so if someone does not feel like talking Lung Qi may be Deficient. This is an internal source for loss of voice called aphonia. Kidney Yin Deficiency can accompany Lung Yin Deficiency to produce dry throat and other hot Yang symptoms.

External invasions act as another disease origin in forms of Wind Heat or Wind Cold, which go directly to the Lungs. In both cases, hoarseness occurs first and leads to a lack of voice. Treatment generally must restore Yin and Lung Qi, while lubricating the vocal cords.

Western medicine concentrates on locating abnormalities of the larynx such as polyps, nodules, and other lesions, or paralysis of the vocal cords. Therapy consists of medication or surgical removal of growths or if needed mechanical maintenance of an open airway.

In consideration of the two basic principles of evaluation— structural pathology and abnormal energy—we discover overlap of abnormal tissues and conditions. Likewise, every disease has details in these two categories. Knowledge of both brings deep insight for effective diagnosis and corrective treatment.

Side-by-side comparisons of Western and Chinese medical concepts certainly broaden a comprehensive outlook on health and disease. Difficulties can arise when a conditioned mindset in anatomy and physiology tries to understand energy systems based on the Chinese manner of interpretation. However, continued exposure will breed familiarity.

(See Laryngitis)

Weight Gain

When I lived and studied in China, I observed that obesity was not as serious a concern as in the United States. I also observed the exuberant activity displayed in daily life. At that time, private automobiles were rare, but buses, taxis, motorcycles, and bicycles dominated the streets. On the sidewalks were masses of walkers, young and old. The expression "a sea of people" now made sense to me. There were occasions where I had to navigate a space for myself after I crossed a street.

Actually, crossing a street required a skill. You never ran, but walked steadily with constant awareness, allowing a group of bicycles to pass before you, or a bus behind you. Vehicles obeyed the red and green lights, but not always the pedestrians.

The point of describing all this on-the-street liveliness, shows continuous bodily activity by human beings, more compact and numerous than I have ever seen, even in New York City. Besides the walkers, huge numbers of bicycle and motorcycle riders abounded, who exerted a lot more vim and vigor than the car drivers.

I saw many things on the streets of China, but I did not see obesity. Still, on occasion, some weighty people did pass by. On closer observation I found that they were firm and not flabby. The latter seems to be an American trait.

It is well known that exercise reduces weight and helps maintain a fine physique. When I travel, I enjoy exploring new territories by foot. So if you need a pleasant way to lose pounds, take a trip and do a lot of walking.

Obesity is a greater concern in the West than the East. We continue to develop new ways to diet, to perform exercise and undergo weight reduction surgery, i.e., gastric bypass. Yet, acupuncturists can offer sought after assistance. Three major categories of evaluation and treatment apply. One deals with food cravings, the second with digestive irregularities and the third for retention of Dampness. Overlapping conditions and therapies often are needed. Different acupuncture offices may vary in their approach. For example, I take into account emotional states, when relevant.

Food addictions demand needling to stop feeding one's mouth or stomach. The ear commonly lends itself for the purpose. Considered an extension of the brain, it sends messages. Points for addiction, the stomach and digestive organs, and relaxation are easily activated. A type of 'press pin' embedded in a waterproof patch, stays in place for continued simulation.

Different needle combinations regulate digestion. Stagnation poses a problem, which responds to quickening its energy and draining off excesses. Some people carry surplus weight in their abdomen. Selected acupuncture points handle the protrusion, which flattens in time.

When not due to gluttony or metabolic weakness, Chinese medicine says look for areas of water retention. Dampness or Heavy Dampness in the form of Phlegm stays put and brings on obesity. A dysfunctional Organ that allows this is the Spleen, which has the responsibility to eliminate abundant fluids. Treatment focuses on the Qi system of Spleen.

Herbal remedies have used processed plants from the sea or

lakes. Energy in the plant holds back superfluous water that could harm the essence of the vegetation. In the human body, it acts in like manner, to restrain the weight-producing Dampness.

A mixed application as indicated of walking exercise, reducing food cravings, regulating the digestive Organs, reducing retained Dampness and strengthening the emotions should achieve a desired effect. In China, many people also do Qigong or Tai Chi Chuan and the population consumes huge amounts of rice and green tea. That was a major part of my diet when I lost weight.

(See Addiction)

Chapter 12
Basic Medical Principles: West and East

So far, discussion has compared Western medicine to Chinese medicine. For simple, but in depth explanations, let's go back to the basics, the fundamental differences between the directions taken by Western civilization and Chinese culture. Both reflect their own forms of thinking that advanced their ways of life, including health practices.

One of my distinguished acupuncture instructors, Dr. Ralph Alan Dale, emphasized the effects on humanity from certain brain functions. Historically, Western nations have conquered and enslaved many foreign cultures to build empires, i.e., Babylonian, Egyptian, Greek, Roman, and British. Cultures blended. This manipulation of human lives shows activity of the left brain. Theories evolved in regards to two sides of the brain, the left and right, and crossover controls. But with few exceptions in the West, religious beliefs of old and ancient languages—written and spoken—and social codes have all been integrated, suppressed or eliminated.

Medical approaches follow, as we wage war and try to conquer and destroy the enemy disease. Armed with antibiotics, surgical excision knives, radiation and chemotherapy, we must kill the evil germs and cut out the detrimental body parts. Diagnostic methods improve to find the culprits through X-ray, MRI, biopsy, and internal examination. As a result, valuable health services within this framework cure disease and repair injury

Another direction replaces what the body can no longer produce, such as insulin in diabetes and blood cells in anemia. Organs are also transplanted in cases of failed function. Overall, it's a matter of controlling nature.

In the past two thousand to four thousand years, China engaged in its share of warfare, but not with other nations. Most fighting took place among people of the same Chinese heritage. Eventually unified, it became unconquerable. When the Mongolians invaded and ruled, more recently in 1215, they were absorbed by the civilized life of their Chinese captives, after a few generations. Foreign colonies set up governing administrations, but not in the central mainland.

Chinese medicine developed from antiquity, without the threat of being dominated by a different ethnic group. Relaxing their left brain of conquest and defeat, they allowed the right brain to take over. In doing so, sensitivity to the forces of nature developed. An intuitive insight grew, observing seasonal changes and how the world balances itself from extremes. Health likewise meant living in harmony with nature. If ill balanced, someone's own energy restored normalcy. Chinese medicine leaned toward the personal experiences and feelings of patients.

The West pursued visualization of abnormalities. In the course of medical history, the microscope gained much usage. One could actually see arrangements of cells in human tissue and disease-producing microbes. Breakthrough discoveries came about thanks to the microscope. And yet, China advanced and gave humanity effective methods to diagnose and treat without the microscope. They applied their expertise in energy.

Yin and Yang

If you understand the concept of Yin and Yang, you will understand the depths of Chinese culture, and the pattern of existence in all its formations and dimensions. It is the universal pattern of duality where everything is paired with an opposite; cold with hot, dark with light, damp with dry, and certainly female with male. All of Chinese Medicine uses Yin and Yang.

The Yin-Yang relationship changes constantly, observed when Yin night goes through phases to become Yang day. There is always a little Yin in Yang and a little Yang in Yin. The goal of health maintenance strives for balance as best possible.

Of major significance is the seesaw phenomenon. Picture two children on a seesaw in a playground. While one goes down the other goes up and vice versa. The same thing happens with Yin and Yang. As Yang descends, Yin ascends. It's the same with disorders of Organs. For example, Deficient Moist Lung Yin produces a Dry Yang unproductive cough, fever, and bronchitis. To remedy, acupuncture or herbs strengthens the Yin. Another case in point is Deficient Kidney Yang. Since Kidney controls the skeletal system and regulates the Heart, symptoms may include arthritis and heart disorders.

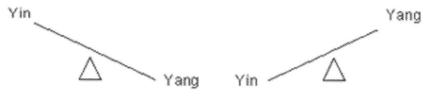

Yin or Yang can dominate and suppress its partner. A preponderance of Yang found in Stomach Fire Blazing causes a hot burning sensation that overpowers the Yin. Treatment concentrates on eliminating the Fire.

Disease-producing Elements have Yin or Yang qualities. Regularly the condition is named as part of the Syndrome such as Damp Heat in the Spleen, Cold Dampness in the Large Intestine or Stirring of Liver Wind.

Qi and Blood

Qi is defined as energy. Not an exact translation from the Chinese, but it is the best we can do to interpret the invisible force. As an active power, Qi has Yang qualities, yet at times it becomes stored. Many categories of Qi exist. Some diseases arise from Qi Deficiency.

Blood houses a type of Qi called Nutritive Qi, which in turn propels its sheltering Blood. They move together and help one another. Certain Syndromes depict Deficiency or Stagnant Blood, in which treatment uses Qi to replace or activate Blood.

$$\frac{Blood}{Qi} \frac{}{Blood}$$

Organs: West and East

Organs have specific anatomical functions. However, our

conventional science of medicine also emphasizes shape, size, and weight (anatomical normalcy), in contrast to Chinese medicine, where Organ energy is of primary concern. For instance, consider the heart. Both schools of medicine agree on its role in blood circulation, but the Chinese also understand it as the home for the Mind. Yet Western medicine has come to recognize connections of mental stress on the heart. In all Organs, acupuncture conditions of Excess, Deficiency, Yin and Yang occur.

Energy activities of Organs assume local and distant duties. Some may overlap functions as defined by Western medicine; nevertheless, the job of Organ Qi is far-reaching.

<u>Heart</u>

Governs Blood and Blood Vessels

Houses the Mind and Spirit

Opens to the tongue and governs speech

<u>Pericardium</u>

Encompasses and protects the Heart

Removes Excesses from the Heart

Involved in mental disorders as is the Heart

Works with Kidney Yang Qi

<u>Lung</u>

Governs Qi and respiration

Rules the exterior surface and Protective Qi that surrounds the body

Regulates water passages

Controls skin and hair

Opens into the Nose

Similar to Western medicine's physiological understanding of the relationship between the heart and lung, the energies of both these organs work together. Heart governs Blood, and Lung governs Qi, and therefore a dependency exists between the two.

<u>Kidney</u>

Stores Essence, the Inherited Qi

Handles birth, growth, reproduction and development

Controls the skeletal system and produces Marrow

Governs water

Holds Qi from the inhaled Breath of Lung

Balances Heart

Powers up Lung and Spleen

Manifests in the hair

Opens into the Ears

Notice some of the relationships among Organs. The Kidney adjusts the Heart and activates Lung and Spleen.

<u>Liver</u>

Stores Blood

Maintains even flow of Qi

Manages muscles, tendons and ligaments

Shown in the nails

Opens at the eyes

<u>Spleen</u>

Transports and transforms food products

Makes and keeps Blood in Vessels

Keeps Internal Organs in place

Governs muscles in the four limbs

Revealed in the lips

Opens to the mouth

Regarding Blood, the Spleen makes it, the Heart governs it and the Liver stores it. This illustrates a functional Qi integration where Organs work together.

<u>Stomach</u>

Center for nourishment

Digests food

Operates closely with the Spleen

Stomach and Spleen are the core for Acquired Qi

<u>Small Intestine</u>

Separates reusable fluids from fluids to be removed

Absorbs nutrients

Adds to the quality of Blood

Associated with urinary and excretory elimination

<u>Bladder</u>

Produces and removes urine

Works with Kidney energy

<u>Large Intestine</u>

Transforms and excretes waste

Absorbs fluids

<u>Gall Bladder</u>

Stores and secretes bile

Connects psychologically to decision making and judgment

Has a close relationship to the Liver

<u>Triple Burner</u>

The Triple Burner consists of three body sections that function as one Organ of different energies. The chest belongs to the Upper Burner, which contains the Lung and Heart. The Middle Burner holds digestive actions of Spleen, Stomach and Gall Bladder. Kidneys, Liver, Intestines and Bladder are found in the Lower Burner for purposes of elimination and reproduction.

Activities of the Triple Burner reveal the entire process of digestion. In addition, it provides the physiological means to combine

Acquired Qi with Inherited Qi that then circulates. Another offering allows Organ Qi to link with Organ Channels.

Knowledge of Organs

Beyond the above, Organs have additional roles. For instance, the Stomach and Spleen have a hand in vaporizing fluid. If excess dampness accumulates in the Lung, the acupuncturist may want to strengthen the Lung. But using knowledge of the Spleen's ability to remove congested moisture will bring about a better result.

Acupuncture is amazingly flexible; needling can be added as needed. Perhaps a fever with stuffed nostrils complicates the Lung disorder. Treatment to reduce the heat then requires extra needles. The same holds true to clear the nose.

Another example concerns a problem of the eye or sight. Dryness, tearing, spots before the eye, or blurry vision all receive help through acupuncture. Aware that the Liver opens at the eyes, the well-trained acupuncturist will also use Liver energy for the therapy.

The greater the familiarity in the workings of Organ Qi, the more successful will be the outcome. This applies to both treatment and evaluation. Symptoms are compiled in a Syndrome of one or two Organ abnormalities. A selection of acupuncture points is made based on the direction to cure the disorder. Perhaps an Organ Yin needs heightening, or Excess Damp Heat must be drained, or the body calls for replacement of Blood and Qi.

Methods of acupuncture differ widely, especially with newer applications that developed in various regions of the world. I have found unique routines even between Chinese provinces. Dissimilar acupuncture practices, based on the same principles, can all be correctly used.

Five Elements

The Five Elements are understood in the context of the Cycle of Creation. In a clockwise rotation starting with Wood, Wood burns to Fire, whose residue becomes Earth, from which we extract Metal, allowing openings for Water to nourish the Wood trees. This concept is as deeply embedded in Chinese culture as are principles of Yin and Yang.

Seasons follow the Cycle. Spring blossoms with plant life of Wood. Summer has the heat of Fire and Late Summer maintains the Earth's growth. Autumn dries and draws out for harvest, and Winter Waters replant for a renewal of seasons.

An application of acupuncture also works with the Five Elements, which organizes the Organs. This shows how Organs function together and how Qi rotates.

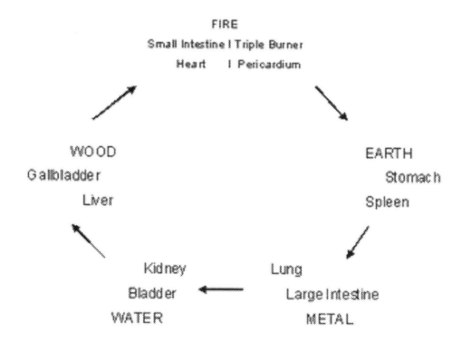

Notice that pairs of Organs fit into the Elements. The Organ pairs are Yin and Yang partners, Yin on the inside and Yang at the outer. They balance one another.

In clockwise fashion, a parent Organ provides energy to a child Organ. For instance, Kidney gives to Liver. If Liver has a Deficiency, acupuncture helps the transfer from Kidney. In another system, every other Organ is controlling or is being controlled. Thus Kidney controls Heart, which controls Lung, which controls Liver, which controls Spleen, which controls Kidney. In a case where the Heart (symbolic of Fire) suffers from excess Heat, acupuncture needling stimulates the Kidney (symbolic of Water) to cool the Heat. Treatments are based on an initial evaluation. When the Organ energy runs like clockwork, usually there are no disorders.

Six Miscellaneous Organs

Less actively involved, these serve more as areas of storage. The designations are Brain, Marrow, Bone, Uterus, Blood Vessels, and Gall Bladder, which has two roles, one to secrete bile and the other, to retain bile.

Meridians, Channels, Pathways

Qi energy passes throughout the body in connecting networks. The original translation of these traveled courses was Meridian, like lines on a globe. With the realization that they have dimension, the word Channel has gained usage. In essence, they are pathways for energy, not to be confused with nerves or blood vessels.

Most branch off Organs, six Yin Meridians off six Yin Organs, and six Yang Meridians off six Yang Organs. It must be remembered that the Fire element contains two pairs of Yin-Yang Organs. They relate directly to their respective Meridian, but some also to the emotions, mind, and spirit. The Stomach Channel extends from the face to the foot. Certain needling of the Channel near the toes treats indigestion but also drains head sinuses. Furthermore, it helps problems on the foot itself. At times, only the Channel remains afflicted and not the Organ.

Energy moves through these attached Channels, each having dominance during a two hour period in a twenty-four hour day. For example, the Liver Meridian exhibits major influence between 1 a.m. and 3 a.m., and the Lung between 3 a.m. and 5 a.m.

Eight Extra Meridians do not stem from Organs; instead they hold reserves of Qi used when needed for deficiencies. Then there are multiple connections with intersections. This large, encompassing complex functions as a means to transport energy and maintain life.

Acupuncture Points

Stimulation at certain points on the body will manipulate energy in an established direction. Needling skills will strengthen, sedate, disperse, and perform many other tasks. Points usually, but not always, belong to a meridian. The stimulation performed by a needle, responds also to a stimulus of pressure, heat, cold, and electric current.

A significant application grew when the Organ Cycle principle was superimposed on the order of Meridians. The result is in an exact science, designating the action of specific points in regulating Qi. By its standard, detailed assessments of diseased energy are made.

Causes of Disease

Some causes in Chinese medicine resemble those in Western medicine to include injury, poison, insect and animal bites, and exhaustion. The big difference appears by China's attention to energy. All types of infliction involve Qi disturbances.

Congenital problems relate to Inherited Qi. Invasions of Wind, Cold, Heat or Damp, at first upset the exterior and then may penetrate deeply into the body. Internally, prolonged negative emotions do their damage, e.g., anger on Liver, hysteria on Heart, worries on Spleen, grief on Lung, and fear on Kidney. Other internal pathologies include Heat, Wind, Phlegm, Stagnation, and Blockages.

Treatment Directly Follows Diagnosis

Frequent examinations consist of taking the pulse, looking at the tongue, checking the complexion and questioning the patient.

A determination can then be made of one's condition, healthy or otherwise, in regard to the status of Organs, Channels, Circulation, Pathogenic Factors, Excesses, and Deficiencies.

A woman in her early twenties with a pensive personality complains of stabbing pains in her stomach, plus nausea and gas. Her pulses feel wiry and choppy, and her tongue appears dark with an oily coating. A yellowish complexion accompanies an anorexic body type.

The acupuncturist makes a diagnosis for a Syndrome of Stagnant Stomach Qi and Congealed Stomach Blood. Immediately, acupuncture needling moves the Stagnation, strengthens the Stomach and regulates Blood.

I must mention that Chinese herbal medication works along the same lines as acupuncture. Pulse examination leans more toward disharmony in the Triple Burners, but the evaluation is equivalent. Remedies taken by mouth eliminate the Stasis, normalize the Stomach and related Organs, and motivate Blood Circulation. Herbs also treat every ailment cared for by acupuncture.

Western medicine's diagnostic data of laboratory studies, X-rays, scans, and biopsies provide important information. However, routines of Traditional Chinese Medicine give the most essential guidelines for effective needling or herbs. In the stomach pain case, our conventional medicine would probably come up with a diagnosis of gastric ulcer or anorexia, which would not furnish a complete basis for Chinese therapy.

Chapter 13
Implementation of Acupuncture

How do we adopt the benefits of acupuncture into our healthcare system? First we must understand the pros and cons of Chinese medicine and patient acceptance. Actually, at present, a fairly large segment of the population in the United States approves of this alternative. Yet many more people could be helped with acupuncture, not to replace Western medicine, but through coexistence. The two medical professions, Western and Chinese, could harmoniously provide their different approaches to diagnostics and therapeutics, each benefiting from the knowledge of the other.

Between 85% and 90% Favorable Results

No form of medicine achieves a 100% cure rate. Good medicine will be reflected in favorable outcomes. Now favorable may not signify a cure, but may indicate control of a disease process, lasting relief or added strength for a disorder needing future reinforcement.

I attempt to cure and, like many other practitioners, feel badly when one is not achieved. In my practice, I see a diversity of ailments and degrees of severity; and a few come in for energy balance and well care. I have calculated that between 85% and 90% of my patients attain favorable results. That means a small number do fall short of our expectations. Worsening of conditions and ill effects remain extremely rare. Much depends on what I have to work with; weakened, lethargic conditions may seem hopeless, but some patients do respond.

A Lot More Than Nerves, Pain Management, and Placebo Effects?

In dealing with medical matters, doctors use what they have learned. Western-trained physicians apply their knowledge of anatomy, biochemistry, and psychology to treat the sick. Likewise, acupuncture practitioners apply their knowledge of body energy to correct unhealthy circulation and conditions.

Nerves

Nerves form a system of connecting fibers throughout a body that conduct impulses to and from the spine and brain. Some nerves, but not all, follow acupuncture Channels. A more subjective medicine, acupuncture relies on a patient's feelings and physical abilities, based on a recounting of their personal experience. Actions of nerves and Qi appear to correlate and overlap, but in reality, differ widely. Along a Qi Meridian, points perform actions established on a pattern of energy flow. The science of neurology is not applicable.

Take for example a powerful Meridian on the upper extremity. Like eleven other Meridians, it contains a Source point, an area of strengthened capability. Needle stimulation here expels pathogenic elements. It also induces delivery when a woman is in labor. This point, therefore, is contraindicated during pregnancy, except at childbirth.

A nearby point on the same Meridian, about an inch away, safely and comfortably relieves nausea in pregnancy. In fact, I routinely needle this point for morning sickness. However, to try and explain the phenomenon by nerve action makes little sense, but familiarity with energy function clarifies everything. Each point carries out unique actions in the manipulation of Qi.

The Source point activates a dynamic force as shown on a chart of energies. According to the sequence of flow, the nausea point fits the qualities of sedation and suppression. Channel strength allows only enough Qi to control morning sickness. Specific physiological responses from certain needle stimulation follow an exact foundation.

Frequently, I use scalp acupuncture, which affects the brain and nervous system. People may say, "Ha! You work on nerves". Not true, I first maneuver energy, which more importantly, manipulates Qi, to correct the affliction. The brain and nervous system are influenced secondarily.

Pain Management

Acupuncture does relieve pain. You can sedate sensations and even anesthetize a part of the body. Often acupuncturists receive referrals when pain medications or physical therapy remain ineffective. From chronic injuries, disease, or surgical complications, all sorts of discomfort may persist. Impairment to structure also impairs energy.

Chinese medical principles address conditions of pain in three kinds of disturbances within Qi and Blood Circulation. One occurs due to obstruction such as Cold or Heat Blockages; another arises

185

from Stagnant Qi, the other from Congealed Blood. Pain is a symptom of an underlying energy disruption. Knowing the type and origin of the pain assists in its elimination.

Placebo Effects

A placebo (an inactive substance) gives relief if the recipient believes it will. That is called the placebo effect. Often it is employed in controlled testing of drugs. One group receives the actual medication and another, the placebo. Comparison of outcomes tells of the drug's efficacy.

Many think acupuncture operates through a placebo effect, but nothing can be further from the truth. Progress over thousands of years has put no importance on suggestion or the premise that you must believe in it for it to work. In fact, when Chinese doctors were first exposed to placebo studies, they found it unethical. They said you should just treat the patient and not play mind games.

Controlled studies in the United States consist of 2 groups. One group receives acupuncture on indicated points for their specific ailment, and the other just random insertions. Results show a much higher degree of relief among those who were treated by prescribed points according to acupuncture standards of care.

Since this type of research is part of the American health system, volunteers will continue to participate. Findings I'm sure will always reveal the general effectiveness of acupuncture therapy.

Changing Attitudes
The Board of Health

While searching for improved methods of medicine, I took an interest in acupuncture when diplomatic relations were opened with China in the early 1970's. I already had a practice in foot surgery since 1968. Hungry for knowledge, I attended every accessible course in subjects related to acupuncture, while I managed a busy office and became active in my local community. The mayor of the city, a patient and friend, appointed me as a member to the city's Board of Health. In time, I was elected chairperson of the Board for two terms.

During this period I invited an acupuncture physician from China to join my practice as my mentor. We agreed he would practice acupuncture and teach me Traditional Chinese Medicine. Historically, one-on-one teacher-student instruction was the norm. Together we established an acupuncture center.

For reasons I did not totally understand, part of the Board of Health wanted me to close the acupuncture facility. One member tried to convince me that acupuncture did not work. A medical director of the city said he liked medicine practiced the way it was and there should be no changes. Also, to maintain my position as chairman, I must discontinue the acupuncture. Soon, the local medical association called and said if I continued the acupuncture center, I must resign my chairmanship. I explained how acupuncture could help the sick. The importance is not to help the sick, he replied, but to be congruent—do your surgery, and prescribe your narcotics, but be congruent.

The mayor was contacted to influence me, although he made it clear that his wife was a satisfied acupuncture patient. Despite all the controversy, I completed my term in office, keeping the acupuncture center open. It successfully served the city. One doctor left the Board, who said he would not be part of a group whose chairman was associated with acupuncture.

The House Visit

Early in my career change as an acupuncturist, a patient called regarding her husband who lay unconscious in bed. I arrived at her home and found a visiting nurse was present. To revive the patient, I activated the Inherited Qi (the Essence) using acupuncture technique and herbal heat (moxa) stimulation.

Suddenly the man opened his eyes and shouted he was hungry and thirsty and wanted whiskey. The nurse was so appalled at this brought-back-to-life happening that she reported me to her supervisor. Her complaint was based on the fact that I treated this unconscious patient without his consent, though the wife consented and they were both patients in my practice. Of course, the supervisor disregarded the unwarranted accusation

Since then, much progress has been made. I lecture at nursing schools, medical organizations, and hospitals. By patient request, I provide acupuncture services in the hospital. Nursing students spend time in my office to observe. A different attitude toward acupuncture has evolved both within the general public as well as in conventional medical institutions.

Educational Backgrounds

China offers every type of medicine in its hospital settings. Medical schools there teach a full spectrum of courses from anatomy, physiology, and pathology to energy dimensions, herbs and acupuncture. Schools are affiliated with hospitals for clinical studies, like in the United States, where students rotate through all clinics, but that also include acupuncture, herbal medicine, and Chinese massage.

In the United States, practitioners who use acupuncture come from widely dissimilar backgrounds. A large number work exclusively in Chinese medicine, while others include it as an added modality. It has proven helpful for anesthetists, psychiatrists, and other medical specialists. Acupuncture courses have gained significance in the educational curriculum for chiropractic and naturopathic physicians.

Ear (auricular) acupuncture sets standards for reversing drug addiction. Trained nurses and therapists now apply the technique. The ear presents itself as a micro-acupuncture system. This means that the entire body is reflected there in miniature, with points for needling. The foot is also a micro-system. Reflexology serves as an example where manual pressures on areas of the foot will treat a related body part. A number of other micro-systems are located on the head, face, hands, back and front and respond accordingly. I also use auricular acupuncture for addiction problems that include alcohol, smoking, and food. It's thought that the ear projects an extension of the brain.

As the Chinese medicine advisor at a local institute for herbal studies, I teach principles of pulse and tongue examination. Practitioners who treat with herbs perform evaluations similar to those done by acupuncturists.

Another course provided instruction in the application of magnets and special seeds in the ear. At a nearby university, I once instructed students from various undergraduate health courses on the principles of acupuncture. This one semester, two credit, course did not teach needle insertion, only medical standards and acupuncture philosophy. Actually, I have been an instructor or guest lecturer at every college and university in my area.

Across the country, students from acupuncture schools graduate after two, three or four year of study. Requirements to practice vary from state to state. Some schools confer master degrees and a few award doctorates. Since differences exist in methods of acupuncture, one finds distinctions, depending on the school. They may emphasize Traditional Chinese methods, or Japanese techniques, or the Five Elements. Whatever the focus, a great deal of acupuncture is performed in the United States with the resulting benefits experienced by many people.

Progress continues in spite of challenges. The State of Connecticut, where I live and practice, greatly opposed acupuncture, and I have had to defend its use through the years. Confidently, I founded the State Acupuncture Association and a related agency for board certification. China's Ambassador to the United Nations came to New Haven as our guest speaker for the Association's inception. All this helped in the establishment of the profession.

To Whom Do You Go?

Acupuncture is widely available, but where do you go? Most of my new patients contact me by referral, from their family, friends, workplace, or other health professionals. I advertise in the yellow pages and have a Web page. At times, someone will notice my office sign and just walk in for an appointment. But overall, referrals account for most of my practice.

If it's your first time seeking acupuncture, and searching for help with a specific disorder, use the phone book. Question those listed regarding their experience in the evaluation and treatment of your ailment. Of course, acupuncture diagnoses differently than Western medicine, so an explanation of the symptoms would be helpful. Familiarity with and working knowledge of a disease through acupuncture has more importance than credentials in other fields.

Acupuncturists are not all the same. Our training varies within

America and from other countries. One method is not necessarily better than another. Though they differ, they still succeed. In the Chinese hospital, I observed a well-known physician who administered a small number of needles for each case; four, five, six or seven. The "Three Needle Technique" also serves as an established routine. Then I viewed the insertion of multiple needles. What's truly remarkable is that all techniques work well.

The development of acupuncture expertise stands apart, and as previously mentioned, differs depending on the training of the practitioner. One of my patients has an ongoing intestinal problem. She used to spend winters in Florida and asked me if I could recommend an acupuncturist there to continue her therapy. I gave her a name of a prominent practitioner and soon received a call from Florida. It was my patient, who informed me that the referral did not render care for her particular condition. However, I know the acupuncturist is very qualified in other areas.

As Western medicine has grown, specialization has been necessary. A specialist may focus on a system (i.e., cardiovascular, gastroenterology, orthopedics). As in the West, Chinese medicine created specialties, ideally to concentrate on one disease. Using the related energy Channels and Organs, a doctor attends to stroke, cancer, or disabilities called atrophy syndromes. Proficiency in treating the disease group reaches high levels of care. There are also Chinese facilities that specialize in one area of affliction. These hospitals use all available treatments.

In America we have not fulfilled the Chinese plan for diversity, but hospitals have incorporated some acupuncture services. There are limitations. Frequently, the presence of flammable oxygen prevents application of moxa. Feeding and intravenous tubes with other attachments often prohibit needle insertion at indicated acupuncture points.

Currently, my ability to render acupuncture in a hospital setting is generally satisfactory. The patient or family requests my services, usually through the nurse's station. Delayed labor, breech birth, surgical complications, and excessive pain will prompt me to make an in-patient visit.

Health Insurance

The expense of health insurance is a major concern. However, when people fail to obtain help by customary and familiar procedures, they usually do not mind paying a reasonable fee, out of pocket, for an alternative that does provide results. Acupuncture requires no elaborate or expensive diagnostic testing. Through consultation and pulse, tongue, and other routines of physical examination, a good evaluation is had. Supplies of acupuncture needles, alcohol swabs, and perhaps paper drapes, add up to a minimal expense. Include the procedural skills of the practitioner, and cost effective treatments can be delivered.

For my part, I accept coverage in accident cases through a mediator (attorney) and in Workers' Compensation cases. Otherwise, payment is expected at the time of service and the office issues a receipt, showing the diagnostic evaluation and treatment code number. The patient may be able to obtain partial reimbursement from the insurer.

I never refuse treatment based on a person's inability to pay. In a financial hardship, I will accept whatever the patient can afford. All health care professionals deserve payment for their services. However, we must be sensitive to and accommodate those who seek our help. In the state that I practice, Medicare refuses coverage. The elderly frequently are the ones in much need of acupuncture, for whom I extend myself. The same courtesy applies to veterans.

For each selection of medical care by the patient, China's healthcare system requires a co-payment at every visit. The government then pays the remainder. In the acupuncture clinics, I observed very positive attitudes as patients paid their fees, then rested comfortably while receiving needles with other modalities. Routinely suction cupping, electrical needle stimulation, and heat lamps were utilized.

Many came to the clinic from their hospital room and or from their homes. Either way, effective therapy often required two or three sessions a week. Notably, multiple patients were treated at the same time, six to twelve in a room with doctor and nurse assistant—privacy was not an issue. Ailments included stroke, injuries, arthritis, asthmatic respiratory disorders, and many more. Causes of diseases by pathogenic invasions or prolonged negative emotions were assessed and remedied as well, with patients experiencing the healing process.

The acupuncture evaluations dictated the courses of treatment. If an X-ray or lab test was ordered, it added information to the Traditional Chinese Medical diagnosis. However, documentation of progress and patient discharge still relied on tongue and pulse examinations and subjective symptoms.

A section of this institution had an intensive care unit (ICU), a department of surgery and availability of Western drugs. It had every possible medical resource, including Chinese herbs and massage. Nevertheless, everything was well organized, despite the thousands of patients that were treated.

The Future

Acupuncture as a medical science uses inexpensive means for diagnostic evaluation and therapy. Since antiquity, it has effectively corrected physical and emotional problems. It offers cures for diseases not discovered by other forms of medicine. So what prevents a more comprehensive acceptance?

First of all, acupuncture comes from a culture on the opposite side of the globe that we are not familiar with. Principles and standards of operation remain foreign to us. We mistakenly interpret the application by models of our conventional medicine, thinking in terms of nerve blocks, psychology, the mind, and hypnosis.

A major breakthrough will come by learning the basics in everyday English. That is why my explanations employ phrases such as internal environment, polarities of the body, and integration of energy with anatomy and biochemistry. Like wind, you cannot see energy, but you can feel energy and see its powerful influence on the visible.

Answers to our healthcare crisis will emerge from education. Not only for the general public, but also for health professionals and administrators, who can bring about improvements. At times I would meet people interested in my medical services. They followed their inquiries by the statement that they must first ask their doctor. It became difficult to explain that their doctor may know a lot or very little about acupuncture.

I have also encountered opposition to acupuncture for competitive reasons, from both medical offices and pharmaceutical companies. I now see this less and less. For the sake of patient health, we need to respect different approaches. In addition, respect must extend to the choices the public makes.

As doctors have pursued medical and surgical specialties, general practice is on the decrease. The acupuncturist can step into this role to treat almost all problems.

As a growing health profession in the United States, acupuncture has made enormous strides. Always in demand however, is improvement. Although states vary in educational requirements and credentials, I feel a resource center for every acupuncture practitioner in the country should be available. This center would provide diagnostic and treatment information from the most current worldwide sources, translations of new findings from China included.

Also a directory that lists practitioners who have developed expertise in the care of certain diseases would be a valuable tool. Both for purposes of consultation and patient referrals, specialized areas within acupuncture have the potential to cure a multitude of diseases. Organized networking would greatly advance knowledge and its application.

Acupuncture is an example of a holistic and natural field for wellness. It and several other services present reasons for us to expand and incorporate a more active part of alternatives in our healthcare system. Millions would benefit.

Considerations for Acupuncture

- Acupuncture should be available. A number of people have needle phobias, probably due to painful experiences from childhood. Skillful hands, however, administer gentle insertions. Pleasant sensations arise while the body moves through a healing process. Those opposed may eventually accept the procedure, which could correct their disease and save their life.

- As the oldest continually practiced medicine in the world, it has withstood the test of time. Principles of acupuncture have remained the same for millennia, unlike other medical sciences that change constantly. The method of diagnostic interpretation and needle treatment done today correlates with that done three thousand years ago.

- It's safe. Rarely do adverse side effects happen. Sometimes bruising appears but poses no danger. As a rule, after acupuncture, nothing changes or there's improvement, and usually there is improvement.

- Easily performed diagnoses require no complex technologies. A consultation with pulse, tongue, or other types of physical examinations gives sufficient information to identify the disorders or syndromes. Treatment directly follows the findings.

- Causes of disease that are explained by Traditional Chinese Medicine could offer insight into puzzling uncertainties. It's a matter of interpretation of symptoms.

- Patient experience of a disorder often has more importance than the doctor's visual examination. This subjective nature of Traditional Chinese Medicine allows an individual to choose a particular health service.

- Office visit sessions suffice for evaluations and treatments. Usually accomplished within an hour; the initial visit may be longer.

- Acupuncture aims to correct the disorder rather than just relieve symptoms.

- Abundant financial spending for diagnostic testing and drug therapy remains unnecessary. Compared to Western medicine, costs are in the hundreds of dollars not thousands, and savings are in the millions.

- Together Chinese and Western medicine will enhance one another, provide better care and cut costs.
- They each have doctors and therapists and, as separate professions, can maintain their own standards of care.

Chapter 14
Commonly Asked Questions

Chinese Medical Science

Isn't acupuncture based on the secretion of endorphins?

Endorphins are proteins, produced in the brain. They can act to reduce pain. Not a foundation for the application of acupuncture, since acupuncture goes beyond pain relief. It regulates circulation, strengthens disabilities, improves Organ function and corrects many disorders of which pain occurs as a symptom. Needle insertion as a healing mechanism elicits various responses in the body. The stimulation may promote the secretion of endorphins or increase blood cells, reduce blood pressure, balance the digestive system and much more. Acupuncture works through energy.

How do you know where to place the needles?

An acupuncturist must become educated in the complex network of energy flow. Needling of points along Channels produces certain actions on energy. By knowing what the points do, a treatment plan is put into place. Anatomical landmarks serve as a guide to locate the exact area for needle insertion.

I realize that you capitalize words that depict energy involvement of organs, substances, and disease-producing elements. Why do you not capitalize the word energy?

Not an exact translation, but the English word energy serves as a defining term for the Chinese principle of Qi. The concept places Qi as the body's continued life function in movement and protection, derived from a source.

Mindful of the pathogenic invasions of Wind, Hot, Cold, and Damp, where does Phlegm fit in?

In Traditional Chinese Medicine, Phlegm is a heavy Damp causative factor for a group of illnesses. Sometimes visible in the Lungs, but often it cannot be seen, settling as an obstruction in the Heart, Gallbladder, Kidney, possibly arthritic joints, and tumors.

What do you feel for in the pulse and look for on the tongue?

The pulse divides into twelve sections that relate to the twelve Organs of Qi. I search for the qualities of flow such as fast, slow, wiry, scattered, etc. This informs me of disturbances in the body's general energy. Also, specific pathology of each Organ is revealed. The tongue reflects the status of internal Organs. I observe abnormalities by the colors coating, shape, and visible changes that can occur.

Can the complexion be diagnostic?

Yes it can. Similar to the tongue, the color, texture, and creases of the face all reflect conditions of the patient.

199

If acupuncture is as wonderful as you say, why was it not discovered and developed by Western medicine?

The Chinese look at the world differently. It's been said that their unique way of life and health truly preserved their ancient culture. As a people who studied extreme seasonal changes, achieving balance with opposites during the yearly cycle, they concentrated on living in harmony with nature. Sickness is considered the result of disharmony and treatment aims to restore balance. Western medicine, on the other hand, evolved as sciences and therefore diagnoses and seeks to cure ailments generally through a cause-and-effect process by eliminating the pathogenic cause.

Patient Care

How often need I return for treatments?

You will feel the effects of acupuncture and know how much you need. Usually reinforcement after the first visit is necessary and perhaps for a few follow-up visits. If your disorder requires a series of sessions, the frequency will decrease as your condition improves.

Will one visit cure a problem?

Quite frequently it will, for a common cold, indigestion, headache and emotional upset. A misconception involves a disease being treated for years. Then, thinking that upon the initial visit, a cure happens. Sometimes it does, often it does not, but continued acupuncture when necessary, reaches higher levels of healing.

Are there other methods of evaluation besides tongue and pulse?

There are, especially from other countries. Tongue and pulse examinations as China's standard, has continued from ancient times. Japan developed methods from abdominal assessments and energy within Channels. America introduced muscle testing related to Meridians. They are all applicable.

I never got acupuncture but how can someone relax comfortably with all those needles?

Your body cannot heal under stress. Once the insertions are made, you enter a very pleasant, altered state of consciousness that lets your body to restore its own health.

So the body heals itself?

Exactly, acupuncture helps the body to heal itself. In comparison, Western medicine intervenes with drugs and surgery. Acupuncture on the other hand works with the forces of nature.

Pulse and tongue examinations are objective in what the doctor feels and sees, so why do you emphasize the importance of what the patient subjectively experiences?

Much importance is placed on patients' self-description of their problems. Even during treatment in China, the acupuncturist asks what is felt in terms of energy response. Pulse and tongue examinations confirm the subjective symptoms.

Can someone be helped with acupuncture and conventional

medicine at the same time?

Depending on the disorder, the two are often compatible. Conflict may come about as acupuncture attempts to rehabilitate a disability by gently restoring circulation of energy. Therapy that uses strenuous exercises will undo the progress.

Administration

Is acupuncture considered a last resort when all else fails?

It could be considered a first or last resort. Many people will initially consult with an acupuncturist for almost any ailment to include allergies, backache, indigestion, insomnia, migraine headaches and depression. Others not familiar with the therapy will try everything before thinking about acupuncture.

I once asked my associate from China what surprised him most about our medicine. He said he was amazed at the number of follow-up surgeries. A surgeon in a Chinese hospital has but one opportunity to perform an operation. If the desired results are not attained, then other types of non-surgical procedures like acupuncture must be employed. In like manner, I have encountered patients unresponsive to acupuncture. They in turn found cures from pharmaceuticals or other interventions.

It seems that a lack of insurance coverage presents the biggest obstacle to advance acupuncture, is that true?

Not really, as many people are willing to pay a reasonable fee for effective care. Lack of public information, however, on how acupuncture helps a wide range of disorders, is an obstacle.

As acupuncture grows and prospers in the United States, will there still be a need for all our established medical services?

Of course there will. Nothing is replaced, only improved, by using every resource available.

What constitutes the best rapport between acupuncture and our conventional medicine?

I believe the referral system we have among specialties will serve as the best model. One doctor recommends a patient to another for a particular indicated treatment. In regard to acupuncture, it can be accepted as one more specialty.

How can our hospitals incorporate an acupuncture facility?

Very easily, with a room or rooms furnished with physical therapy type of tables, chairs and hangers for clothes. Curtains can serve as separators for privacy. One consultation desk belongs in each room. A tabletop would contain alcohol swabs, cotton tip applicators, boxes of needles and a hazardous waste receptacle. Modalities of suction cups, electric machines, moxa, or heat lamps need a storage area. Add qualified acupuncturists and we're in business.

Chapter 15
In Conclusion

Quality of Life

Acupuncture promotes quality of life at all ages. People may live long, but do they retain vitality and agility? Are they without pain? In China I saw large numbers of elderly briskly walking the streets with a smile. They knew exactly their treatment needs in the acupuncture or massage clinics, and at the herbal pharmacy. These seniors live with a quality of life created by choices. Diagnostic evaluations are performed at each facility, usually by pulse, tongue, and elicitation of symptoms. If sought, Western medical methods could be chosen as well.

Both types of medicine borrow from one another to reach the highest possible competence in patient care. Surgical anesthesia employs acupuncture. Herbs are distilled and the extract administered intravenously or injected into an acupuncture point. Surgery will drain an infected organ that responds neither to herbs or acupuncture. Acupuncture, in turn, aids healing in the postoperative period.

Need exists for every field of medicine. Patients benefit from the availability and choices. The sick strive to restore their health, as effectively and inexpensively as possible. And those in good health must maintain their hardy physical and mental states.

Always Yin and Yang

In a comparative description of therapies, East to West, of significance is that the Chinese view of the world stays based on duality of existence—Yin and Yang. In their observation of nature, they found this dichotomy everywhere. Accordingly, it serves as the infinite pattern and basis for understanding health and disease. Herbal remedies, massage therapy, and acupuncture all use it in their respective routines of diagnosis and treatment.

Chapters in this book made analogies between Western and Chinese medicine. We covered basic scientific principles, interpretations of diseases and methods of treatment. In common, both strive to establish an accurate diagnosis and a plan to treat the disease. Each has its concerns for injuries, toxins, and emotional stress.

Contrasts appear when one type of medicine focuses on normal and abnormal structure, chemistry, and behavior, as well as infection-producing microorganisms. The other concentrates on healthy and afflicted energy, evaluated by signs and symptoms. Pathogenic, atmospheric invasions and prolonged negative emotions are understood as causes.

In general, Western medicine attempts to remove or suppress the source of illness, with drugs, surgery, and other interventions. Weaknesses gain strength by nutritional and rehabilitative therapy.

Chinese medicine focuses on balancing harmful conditions. If too hot, cool it down; if too cold, warm it; if too dry, moisten it; if too damp, dry it; if there is an excess, reduce it; if deficient, replenish it; if blocked, clear it; if stagnant, activate it.

Through the knowledge of every health resource, we can compare and select what best meets our needs. Our individual life-styles, combined with daily routines, are grounded in feelings of well being and active abilities. These differ from person to person. Therefore, in addition to the medical help provided in our communities, we must also become self-guided.

A huge library of acupuncture references resulted from thousands of years of progress. Ongoing research, especially in China, expands the massive knowledge. Patient cases in English, documented in the American Journal of Acupuncture, were published from the 1970s to the 1990s. The Journal of Chinese Medicine, which I have subscribed to for three decades, contains case studies and up-dated translations from Chinese to English. The means for extensive learning and application is available to us.

Increased Patient Care, Decreased Expense

The most effective solution for our healthcare system centers on high quality of care with low costs. A medical budget that coexists with acupuncture will succeed. Patients familiar with the various health services are able to choose what best meets their needs.

Diagnosis and treatment reduce expenses. Routines of Traditional Chinese Medicine take little time to make a diagnosis. If the evaluation requires additional information, selected laboratory and X-ray studies are always available.

Acupuncture therapeutic procedure requires a minimal amount

of supplies. Easily performed by small numbers of medical personnel, so many patients could benefit in a day.

Bibliography

Bensky, Dan and O'Connor, John. *Acupuncture, A Comprehensive Text*. Chicago: Eastland Press, 1983.

Bensky, Dan and Gamble, Andrew. *Chinese Herbal Medicine Materia Medica*. Seattle: Eastland Press, 1993.

Berkow, Robert (ed). *The Merk Manual,* 18th ed. Rahway, NJ: Mark Research Laboratories, 2006.

Byers, Dwight. *Better Health with Foot Reflexology*. St. Petersburg, FL: Ingham Publishing, 1983.

Chirall, Ilkay. *Cupping Therapy.* London: Harcourt Brace and Company Limited, 1999.

Dale, Ralph. *The Origins and Future of Acupuncture*. N. Miami Beach, FL: Dialectic Press, 1982.

Deadman, Peter and Al-khafaji, Mazim. *A Manual of Acupuncture*. East Sussex, England: Journal of Chinese Medicine Publications, 1998.

Dunbar, William and Chelnick, Robert and Plovanich, Daniel and Fian, Robbee. *Zang Fu Principles and Diagnosis*. Twin Lakes WI: Clear Lakes Publishing, 1997.

Fleischman, Gary, 1996. Possibilities for the Treatment of Cystic

Fibrosis with Acupuncture and Chinese Herbs: Theory and Case Study. *American Journal of Acupuncture* Vol: 24 pages 135–142.

Fleischman, Gary. *Acupuncture: Everything You Ever Wanted To Know*. Barrytown, NY: Barrytown, LTD. Station Hill Openings, 1998.

Frank, Benjamin. *Dr. Frank's No-Aging Diet*. New York: The Dial Press, 1976.

Jin, Yu. *Obstetric and Gynecology in Chinese Medicine.* Seattle: Eastland Press, 1998.

Kaptchuck, Ted. *The Web That Has No Weaver*. New York: Congdon & Weed, 1983.

Liu, Guohui. *Warm Diseases A Clinical Guide*. Seattle: Eastland Press, 2001

Lu, Henry. *Chinese Herbal Cures*. New York: Sterling Publishing Co., 1994.

Lukas, Richard. *Secrets of the Chinese Herbalists*. West Nyack, NY: Parker Publishing Company, 1977.

Maciocia, Giovanni. *Diagnosis in Chinese Medicine*. London: Elsevier Limited, 2004.

Maciocia, Giovanni. *The Foundations of Chinese Medicine*. Edinburgh: Churchill Livingstone, 1989.

Ni, Maoshing. *The Yellow Emperor's Classic of Medicine*. Boston: Shambhala Publications, 1995.

Scott, Julian and Barlow, Teresa. *Acupuncture in the Treatment of Children, 3rd ed*. Seattle: Eastland Press, 1999.

Shen, De-Hui and Wu, Xiu-Fen and Wang, Nissi. *Manual of Dermatology in Chinese Medicine*. Seattle: Eastland Press, 1995.

Willcox, Bradley and Willcox, Craig and Suzuki, Makoto. *The Okinawa Program*. New York: Clarkson Potter Publishers, 2001.

Wang, Jo-Yi. *Applied Channel Theory in Chinese Medicine*, Seattle: Eastland Press, 2008.

Zhu, Mingqing. *A Handbook for Treatment of Acute Syndromes by Using Acupuncture and Moxibustion*. Hongkong: 8 Dragons Publishing, 1992.

Index

215